D0242178

Successful Fitness Motivation Strategies

Barbara A. Brehm

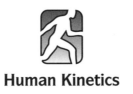

Human Kinetics

Library of Congress Cataloging-in-Publication Data

Brehm, Barbara A.
  Successful fitness motivation strategies / by Barbara A. Brehm.
    p. cm.
  Includes bibliographical references and index.
  ISBN 0-7360-4593-7 (soft cover)
  1. Physical fitness--Psychological aspects. 2. Motivation (Psychology) I. Title.
  GV481.2.B74 2004
  613.7'1--dc22
                                    2004002097

ISBN: 0-7360-4593-7

Copyright © 2004 by Barbara A. Brehm

All rights reserved. Except for use in a review, the reproduction or utilization of this work in any form or by any electronic, mechanical, or other means, now known or hereafter invented, including xerography, photocopying, and recording, and in any information storage and retrieval system, is forbidden without the written permission of the publisher.

Acquisitions Editor: Michael S. Bahrke, PhD; **Developmental Editor:** Renee Thomas Pyrtel; **Assistant Editor:** Ann M. Augspurger; **Copyeditor:** Annette Pierce; **Proofreader:** Joanna Hatzopoulos Portman; **Indexer:** Betty Frizzéll; **Permission Manager:** Dalene Reeder; **Graphic Designer:** Fred Starbird; **Graphic Artist:** Dawn Sills; **Photo Manager:** Kareema McLendon; **Cover Designer:** Keith Blomberg; **Photographer (cover):** © Comstock IMAGES; **Photographer (interior):** all photos © Human Kinetics unless otherwise noted; **Art Manager:** Kelly Hendren; **Illustrator:** Kelly Hendren; **Printer:** United Graphics

Printed in the United States of America   10 9 8 7 6 5 4 3 2 1

Human Kinetics
Web site: www.HumanKinetics.com

United States: Human Kinetics
P.O. Box 5076
Champaign, IL 61825-5076
800-747-4457
e-mail: humank@hkusa.com

Australia: Human Kinetics
57A Price Avenue
Lower Mitcham, South Australia 5062
08 8277 1555
e-mail: liaw@hkaustralia.com

Canada: Human Kinetics
475 Devonshire Road Unit 100
Windsor, ON N8Y 2L5
800-465-7301 (in Canada only)
e-mail: orders@hkcanada.com

New Zealand: Human Kinetics
Division of Sports Distributors NZ Ltd.
P.O. Box 300 226 Albany
North Shore City
Auckland
0064 9 448 1207
e-mail: blairc@hknewz.com

Europe: Human Kinetics
107 Bradford Road
Stanningley
Leeds LS28 6AT, United Kingdom
+44 (0) 113 255 5665
e-mail: hk@hkeurope.com

I dedicate this book with deep appreciation to my parents, Carl and Lois Brehm. Despite your early misgivings about the benefits of physical activity, you have both embraced exercise with open minds. Thanks for everything, even the pink football you gave me for Christmas the year I decided to major in physical education.

Contents

Chapter 4 Developing the Force of Habit   63

Chapter 5 Fostering Positive Exercise Experiences   91

Chapter 6 Working With the Clinical Population: Focus on Ability   113

Preface

After teaching group exercise classes and designing individualized exercise prescriptions for several years, I became fascinated with the adherence enigma. Why was it that despite my dedicated, educated, and energetic cheerleading, a sizable portion of my clients and students dropped out of my class or program after a few months? Was it something about them? Me? Exercise in general?

One class in particular challenged all of my (fairly uninformed) assumptions about which students would be most likely to stay with the class for several months and which could be easily pegged as potential dropouts. The year was 1980, and I was teaching several classes in New York University's brand-new Coles Sports and Recreation Center. One was an aerobics class (we called it aerobic dance back then, and music was supplied by vinyl records) that met at eight o'clock in the morning.

On the first day of class, I greeted my new students cheerfully as they entered the studio. Some bounded in full of energy and enthusiasm. Others looked around tentatively, sizing up the crowd to see if they really belonged, taking their places in the back row, as far from me as possible.

The class was packed that day, but I remember two students in particular. One was fairly young and extremely enthusiastic. After the class she spent quite of bit of time explaining to me her reasons for taking the class and telling me how much she loved my class. I was, of course, soaking up the compliments and congratulating myself on being such a great teacher. I never saw her again.

The other student was a neatly and conservatively dressed woman in her late 30s who was polite but aloof. She rarely smiled, and indeed looked very serious during the workout, in contrast to most of the other students who were grinning and laughing at my jokes. When I engaged her in conversation from time to time (she was always two minutes early for class) she was pleasant but distant. During the three-month session, she never missed a class.

I learned from this experience that, just as you cannot judge a book by its cover, you cannot predict students' adherence from their initial enthusiasm. I realized that I had a lot to learn about exercise adherence, and I grew curious about the many factors that contribute to fitness success.

For the past 25 years I have studied motivation and adherence from both an academic perspective as a professor in the department of exercise and sport studies at Smith College and from an applied perspective as a fitness instructor, personal trainer, and fitness program director. This book has grown out of these experiences. Although solidly grounded in the research literature, it is written from a holistic perspective that incorporates material from a wide range of disciplines and the experiences of the many exercise science and fitness professionals I have had the opportunity to work with over my career.

This book is written for everyone who works to help people design and stick to exercise programs. It will be especially helpful to fitness professionals who want to know how to structure physical activity programs that will lead to success for their clients. This book should be of interest to people working as or studying to become personal trainers or exercise instructors, as well as others working in the fitness center setting. This book is also written for allied health professionals in physical therapy, cardiac rehabilitation, and other situations in which exercise is prescribed for therapeutic purposes. Health and fitness professionals working in community, educational, recreational, and workplace health promotion settings will also find the information in this book helpful.

This book begins with a chapter on the role of the health and fitness professional as motivator, and the importance of good communication skills. Effective communication skills are the foundation of rewarding working relationships between you and your clients. These relationships will increase the likelihood that your recommendations will fit your clients' needs and will lead to exercise programs your clients will be satisfied with. Too often fitness professionals become caught up in the science of exercise prescription before getting a sense of who their clients are and what they might be searching for.

Chapter 2 presents an applied overview of the psychology of behavior change, using the stages of change model to answer two important questions: How do people go about changing their habits, and how can this process allow you to be an effective catalyst? Chapters 3 and 4 get down to business and offer advice for effectively introducing your client to physical activity and setting a direction that is most likely to result in successful adherence. People are most likely to find motivation for physical activity if they engage in programs that hold personal meaning or interest for them. Chapter 5 covers the tried-and-true techniques of behavior modification, as applied to physical activity.

Chapter 6 presents information on motivation in clinical care settings. Chapter 7 presents information on enhancing adherence in group exercise settings, beginning with motivational strategies for group exercise leaders. Chapter 8 covers program strategies for fitness centers. This chapter also presents ideas for reaching a wider and increasingly diverse population, in which many people face significant barriers to physical activity.

Health science research continues to emphasize the importance of regular physical activity for maintaining health and preventing chronic disease. Inactivity is now considered a major risk factor for many lifestyle-related diseases, including heart disease, type 2 diabetes, obesity, hypertension, osteoporosis, and some cancers. Regular exercise slows many of the negative effects associated with aging, reduces stress, and adds life to your years. Yet the cultural forces against becoming physically active have never been stronger. Most occupations have become increasingly sedentary. Labor-saving devices have reduced the caloric expenditure once inherent in house and yard maintenance activities. We don't even need to get out of our chairs to change the channel on the television, or leave the car to open the garage door. Although many of these changes seem small, together they greatly reduce the requirement for daily physical activity. Because little activity occurs as a natural component of daily living, most people can avoid a sedentary lifestyle only by creating opportunities for physical activity. Here again the cultural forces against personal exercise programs are strong. Who has the time? Money? Facilities? Knowledge? Energy? Many people report that regular exercise requires more time and energy than they can spare in their high-stress, fast-paced lifestyles.

The goal of this book is to increase your knowledge of current issues in exercise motivation and adherence so that you can more effectively help your clients negotiate a cultural environment that so often discourages physical activity. As you work to motivate and increase the adherence of the people you work with, you will become more effective as a fitness professional. While increased involvement on your part may initially seem like more work, the more you invest in your skills, the more rewards you will reap. On first appearance, people come to you for exercise advice. But they may also be looking for community and connection, and even meaning, in their exercise experiences. You are not just an exercise scientist; you are a cheerleader, a coach, and a source of inspiration to those around you. As you become more confident and competent in these roles, you will find that you benefit personally from the richer experiences you create for yourself in your work and in your life.

Acknowledgments

Many writers have observed how ideas that turn into a book seem to flow from fingers to keyboard of their own accord. We write acknowledgments because we know that these ideas actually take shape out of our years of reading, studying, researching, listening to lectures, and engaging in conversation. Thus, this book is the product of thousands of thought-provoking interactions with friends, family, colleagues, students, and even those strangers sitting next to me on the airplane.

I am grateful for all of the terrific people I have discussed exercise with over my 30 years in this wonderful field. Leading the list are my colleagues in the department of exercise and sport studies at Smith College: Don Siegel, Jim Johnson, Chris Shelton, Jane Stangl, Lynn Oberbillig, Esther Haskvitz, Tim Bacon, and Jackie Blei. They have always been supportive and inspiring, and because of them I look forward to going to work every day.

Wherever I go I visit fitness centers and talk to owners, staff, and clients about exercise adherence. Thanks to all of you who have taken the time to share your ideas and stories with me.

The Smith Fitness Program for Faculty and Staff is one of my laboratories for exploring exercise adherence. Our department's administrative assistant, Michelle G. Finley, makes sure the program runs smoothly, as do our terrific instructors, Rosalie Constantilos, Lisa Thompson, Craig Collins, and Joan Kosa. My other laboratory is a summer program offered by Smith College Executive Education. I am grateful to director Barbara Rheinhold and program manager Iris Marchaj for their strong support of my work with the women executives who attend this program. Special thanks also go to the hundreds of people I have worked with in these programs over the years.

My family, especially my husband, Peter, has been extremely supportive throughout the writing process. Our sons, Ian and Adam, provide plenty of opportunity for activity so I don't spend all day at the computer. Visiting relatives, including my sister Susan Hall and her family, ask to hear about the book, and provide stories of their own. My father-in-law, Fred Curtis, appears thinly disguised as Bud in chapter 6, and I am inspired to see he still walks every day with his wife (and my mother-in-law), Audrey Curtis. Maybe that is why he is the picture of health at age 91!

Ideas that flow from fingers to keyboard need a publisher to reach their audience, and I am deeply appreciative of the people I have worked with at Human Kinetics. Thanks to Mike Bahrke, Renee Thomas Pyrtel, and Annette Pierce, who turned my pages of manuscript into a real live book.

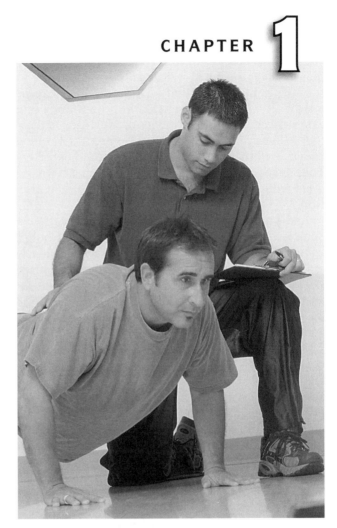

Your Role in the Exercise Adherence Story

Health and fitness professionals are generally a wonderful group. While no two look or act the same, they usually share several qualities. They tend to be high-energy, fun-loving, and dynamic people. Get a group together for a master class or workshop and the studio feels ready to explode with energy. The air becomes charged with exuberance, enthusiasm, and passion for physical activity.

People decide to work in the fitness business for a variety of reasons. Many are seeking an alternative to the daily grind, especially a daily grind that involves sitting at a desk all day. Most have found deep personal rewards in physical activity. They may have excelled at sports or lost weight after years of struggling with their body image. Almost all have experienced the profound sense of well-being and pleasurable relaxation that follows physical exertion. Many routinely enjoy that state of grace known variously as "flow," "being in the moment," or the "exercise high." These experiences are so meaningful, it's no wonder we want to share them with others. If this sounds like you, you are in the right profession.

And your work is needed more than ever! Over the past several decades, the average daily activity level of people in industrialized countries, including the United States and Canada, has declined considerably (Hill and Melanson 1999). This decline in physical activity and the stress that accompanies a sedentary lifestyle have been associated with an epidemic of lifestyle-related illnesses, including depression, anxiety disorders, artery disease, obesity, hypertension, and diabetes (Booth and Chakravarthy 2002).

The human body was made to move. It needs activity to stay healthy as much as it needs air, water, and food. Yet only about 30 percent of adults in the United States meet the Centers for Disease Control and Prevention and the American College of Sports Medicine (ACSM) recommendation of 30 minutes or more of moderately intense physical activity on most days of the week (Booth and Chakravarthy 2002). The solution to this problem is deceptively simple: People need to get moving! Of course, many do try to become more active. They find ways to squeeze exercise into their lives. Some of them are your students, clients, and friends. But because life contains so many obligations that compete with exercise, and because exercise can take much time and effort, it is a difficult habit for many to maintain. Hundreds of studies have monitored the attendance of people who begin an organized exercise program, such as an exercise class or individually prescribed programs of physical activity. In the long run, on average, only about half of the participants will still be involved in the program six months later (Dishman 1994).

Is the class half empty or half full? You could view this 50 percent adherence rate in several ways. Fitness professionals are usually dismayed that they lose half of their students, clients, or members. On the other hand, they could be happy that half manage to stay with the exercise program after six months. And maybe some of the people who drop out continue to exercise on their own; they just can't make it to the gym two or three times a week. Or maybe they will pick it up again next week. This 50 percent rate is much higher than the rate of people who manage to quit smoking in a smoking cessation program or who succeed in overcoming an addiction to drugs or alcohol in a treatment program.

Changing behavior is difficult. Think about behaviors you have tried to modify. Have you ever tried to change your eating habits? Quit smoking? Quit procrastinating and start earlier on writing a term paper or studying for final exams? Keep your desk more organized? Adding exercise to your routine is no different. Many studies have looked at the psychology of behavior change and at factors that increase the likelihood that people will be successful in their behavior change plans, including their attempts to become more active. This book shares the results of this research with you so that you can effectively help people become regular exercisers.

I believe that who you are and how well you work can have a tremendous impact on how successful your clients are in reaching their fitness goals. In this chapter we take a quick look at the concepts of exercise adherence and motivation. Then we encourage you to examine your own professional goals, along with those of your organization if you work in one, to see how these affect your decision to implement new adherence strategies in your work. Next, we examine how your professional and ethical conduct can promote exercise adherence in those with whom you work. We also discuss the importance of good communication skills for working productively with clients and colleagues. Working with clients takes energy, so this chapter concludes with a few words about self-renewal, stress management, and avoiding burnout.

What Is Meant by Exercise Adherence and Motivation?

Adherence is an interesting word. To some it might bring to mind images of bandages or duct tape. But for fitness professionals, adherence refers to the concept of "sticking to," in this case, an exercise program. Exercise adherence is the extent to which people follow, or stick to, an exercise program.

Research on exercise adherence is concerned with how often people engage in physical activity and examines whether or not people stick to the exercise programs they have enrolled in. Because people who drop out of formal programs often become inactive, inactivity and enrollment are closely related. Factors that help people stick to formal exercise programs tend to be similar to factors that increase people's ability to schedule activity into their days; therefore, the research has much to offer. And of course, in our profession we are often concerned with attendance, whether or not people stay with us as their personal trainers, and what percentage of our members renew their memberships. For these reasons, the research on exercise adherence forms the foundation of this book.

The concept of exercise adherence can lead to negative thinking, so you should avoid the term with most of your clients. *Adherence* implies that you are either sticking to the program or you are not. This is dangerous thinking because people tend to give up easily once they label themselves as failing. You have probably known people who are either on a diet (eating in a dangerously restrained fashion) or off their diet (giving in to the cravings created by the restrained eating and consuming everything in sight). In other words, it would probably be more productive to say, "Were you physically active yesterday? What did you do?" rather than, "Did you stick to your exercise program?"

You may hear exercise psychologists using the word *compliance,* another word found in behavior change research. Compliance has even more negative connotations than adherence. Compliance is used primarily in a medical setting, referring to whether or not patients comply with, or follow, doctors' orders. In our field, compliance suggests that clients are passive recipients of an exercise prescription written by an exercise physiologist, and that clients should follow the expert's recommendations. This notion of compliance overlooks the reality that when it comes to increasing physical activity, changing behavior requires extensive involvement and effort on the part of the client. A more productive orientation is this: We, clients and fitness and health professionals, are a team working together to help people become more active. Medical practitioners, too, are starting to view the provider–patient relationship as a collaborative working relationship. People are most likely to be successful in their behavior change efforts when they are extensively engaged in the decisions affecting their lives rather than complying with the recommendations of another person.

When exercise scientists talk about exercise adherence they often discuss the concept of motivation. As fitness professionals we assume that part of our work is to motivate people and to help set up motivational situations (social support, pleasant environments, rewards, and so forth) that increase participation in physical activity.

Motivation is derived from the Latin root *movere*, which means to move. Therefore it is especially meaningful to use the word *motivation* in connection with physical activity. Motives refer to impulses, inner drives, or intentions that cause a person to move, to do something, or to behave in a certain way. Fitness instructors hope that someone who is appropriately motivated will decide to participate in regular physical activity. This is a simplistic assumption, of course, because motivation to exercise changes from moment to moment and competes with motivation to participate in other activities (and inactivities). Even the strongest exercise motivations can quickly fizzle when they run up against complicated real-life situations. Nevertheless, motivation is an important part of the exercise adherence puzzle.

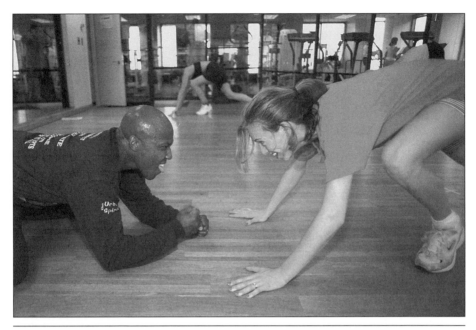

Motivation is a key to exercise adherence, and fitness professionals can be instrumental in helping clients maintain their motivation.

Researchers have spent years trying to figure out what motivates people to get moving. Not surprisingly, they have found that hundreds of factors can help predict whether a person will decide to start participating in regular physical activity. These and other factors also help predict whether they will stick with, or adhere to, their resolutions to become more active.

Exercise Adherence and Career Development

As you begin to choose adherence strategies to implement in your work, think about how these strategies might enhance your personal and professional goals. Before you begin creating new programs or changing the way you do things, you need a clear idea of why you do what you do. It's also important to feel that the work you do each day takes you where you want to go. When we think about adherence-enhancing strategies, we tend to focus immediately on what we can do for others, not on what we want from our jobs. But we can reach out more effectively when we work from the heart and when our daily work is congruent with our short- and long-term career and personal goals. Improving the way you work with clients must be something you do in part for yourself, not just for your clients or for your organization. When you feel motivated, you have more energy and creativity for your work with others.

Instructors in stress management, time management, sport psychology, and leadership often take students on a mental journey into the future. The journey begins by taking time to be alone, turning off the phone, and turning your attention inward. Begin by taking a few deep breaths, closing your eyes, and relaxing your muscles. Imagine yourself at the end of your life, as a very old person. Think back on your life. What have you accomplished? How have you lived? What was important? Think holistically, and include in this meditation not only career goals but also goals for your personal life. Write these thoughts on a piece of paper. You will probably end up with a list of values, events, and accomplishments.

Many find this a stimulating but somewhat daunting exercise. Embedded in this visualization are many big questions: Who are you? What is your purpose in life? What is the meaning of life? What is meaningful and important? What gives you satisfaction and pleasure? What are you doing now to achieve these goals? You will consider these questions throughout your life, and your thoughts will change as time goes by. Even though your ideas will change over the years, your thoughts on these matters will give your life meaning and direction.

After you have looked at the big picture of your life, think about the next five years. What are your personal and professional goals for this period? How will these goals move you toward your lifetime goals? What kinds of activities will help you accomplish these goals? How is what you are doing now helping you toward these goals? Think about how you live. What changes would you like to make? Record your thoughts and ideas about your five-year goals and activities.

Take another moment to think about all the things you do right, and be thankful for the opportunities you have had. Think about an event that made you feel great to be alive. Maybe you received praise for a project well done or a smile from a child you helped. Perhaps you earned a good grade on a project or received a job offer you really wanted. As you remember these events, dwell in the good feelings these memories bring, feeling good about yourself and your life. Keep a mental collection of these positive memories, and draw on them for strength and direction.

Life is never perfect, but full of limitations and constraints within which we must maneuver. We will be most successful if we can live with a sense of humor, gratitude, hope, optimism, and openness to what life brings.

Many writers have compared life to a canoe trip down a river. We cannot change the river, but we can navigate its course with greater or lesser skill. Some decisions take us down a smoothly flowing course, whereas others hang us up in the shallows. Sometimes we run into rapids that require sharp attention. Our values and goals are the tools for navigating our course down this river. We have little control over many parts of our lives, but given our situation and abilities, we can live according to our values and seek to accomplish our most important goals. Our lives can be a path with a heart.

Let's return to the topic of exercise adherence and motivation for physical activity. Did helping people become healthier or more active find its way into your goals? Did you want to increase the productivity of your time spent at work, reaching more people? Did you hope to develop a successful career in the fitness field? If so, then your work in devising adherence strategies for the people with whom you work will take shape relatively easily once you begin to explore alternative ways of working.

Q&A

Q I'm definitely interested in improving exercise adherence at the community fitness center where I work. I am a personal trainer and teach several group exercise classes. But I am running so fast already, I can hardly catch my breath. Help! How can I ever find the time to do one more thing? Some days I am drowning in work.

A Many people feel overwhelmed by their jobs from time to time. Adding one more project is not the answer. Instead, think of how you could work smarter, not harder. As you read this book, you may decide to simply change the way you do something rather than to add additional tasks to your job description. If you decide a new program would be helpful, then you would need to identify a less-helpful program (or two programs?) to eliminate. Talk to coworkers to help you and your organization clarify your priorities, and do the most important things first. If your job seems to be too much, then talk with your supervisor. If you are the supervisor, talk to your peers and think about ways to make your work more manageable.

Exercise Adherence and Your Organization

Some fitness professionals work alone, but most work within some sort of organization. Even those who contract individually with worksites must keep in mind the organization's needs and constraints when designing programs. Now that you have your own goals in mind, consider how they fit into the goals and procedures of the organizations you work in.

As you start thinking about your organization, its mission statement is a good place to start. If you don't know what the mission statement is, ask your supervisor. If your organization doesn't have a mission statement, consider writing one. A mission statement is simply a few sentences that describe the purpose and goals of the organization, sometimes along with its principles and values.

If you have been with your organization for some time, you may have discovered unwritten purposes, goals, and ways of operating. For example, your organization's mission statement may not say anything about making money, but almost every organization operates within some sort of financial constraints. Health clubs may make money by selling memberships; some fitness centers charge for programs. A worksite center may be able to accommodate only a limited number of users. Consider how increasing exercise adherence might enhance (or in some cases hurt) your organization's written and unwritten goals.

Sample Mission Statement: What It Says and What It Doesn't Say

The following mission statement belongs to a small workplace fitness program:

> "Our mission is to provide safe, effective, high-quality, low-cost exercise opportunities for company employees. We strive to provide excellent group exercise instructors and to be responsive to the needs of our participants."

This mission statement is short and sweet. If you were to talk to the program director, you would find out that administering this program is also based on many other principles and constraints, including the following:

- This program must comply with industry standards for safety and injury prevention. Instructors must be certified in their activity and in CPR, and they must be familiar with company emergency procedures.

- Except for the director's position, this program is primarily self-funded; therefore, client fees must cover operating costs. The program consists primarily of group exercise classes. All classes must be as full as possible.

- This program should operate efficiently. Therefore, it is important to retain high-quality instructors in order to reduce the program director's administrative load.
- This program must work closely with the company's department of human resources (HR) so that its activities complement and do not duplicate those offered by HR. This program must also fulfill the perceived needs of the company as stated by HR.

As you think about exercise adherence and motivational strategies that might work for you and your organization, keep in mind your organization's market. What kind of clients does your organization want to serve? What kind of clients are you actually serving? Is your organization interested in expanding, changing, or narrowing its market?

What is your position in your organization? What does "excellent performance" mean for people in your position? Other workers in your organization? How does change occur within your organization? If you would like to implement changes, with whom should you discuss your ideas? Who can help you? How might these changes affect other programs? Whom might this affect? Be sure to include these people in your discussions.

What future trends might affect your organization? Is the population in your area aging? Are economic conditions changing? What organizations compete with you in your market? Will local concerns affect your programming? Are people concerned about the increasing prevalence of obesity in young people? Inadequate requirements for and content of physical education courses in the schools? A need for more opportunities for activity for older adults?

As you think about implementing new strategies for increasing physical activity, keep in mind local organizations with whom you might form a coalition or partnership. Many fitness centers expand their programs and their revenue by working with hospitals, health care providers, schools, senior centers, employers, and even recreational sports leagues.

Your Professional and Ethical Conduct Enhances Exercise Adherence

A seasoned but somewhat cynical exercise program director once made the following observations when asked about the role of fitness professionals in motivating clients and increasing exercise adherence: "There are many things we can do to help make physical activity a quality experience. But even the best instructors in the world will have many clients who quit exercising, no matter what the instructors do. There are just so many other variables involved. On the other hand, a poor instructor can really turn people away. It's kind of depressing if you think about it: A good instructor has limited power, but a poor one can have a huge negative influence."

It is true that poor instructors can turn people away. But this director may be underestimating his good instructors. One might argue that good instructors, personal trainers, and other fitness professionals, while unable to actually make clients physically active, can have a significant influence on many people. They can design effective exercise programs and give sound exercise advice. Their attitudes and behaviors certainly affect whether or not a person decides to return to their facilities or classes, or to choose them as personal trainers. They can train clients in strategies that support behavior change and increase exercise adherence in many positive ways.

Most health and fitness professionals have a fairly good idea of what it means to be a *professional* fitness professional. A good way to think about professionalism in your current career is to think about provider–client relationships in general. Put yourself into the client or patient position and think about what creates a good relationship with someone you have gone to for help. Take a minute to recall both negative and positive experiences you have had with practitioners in the helping professions. Think about the worst and the best interactions you have had as a student, client, or patient; also consider the worst and best interactions you've had with fitness professionals, health care providers, teachers, counselors, and other people you have sought advice from.

Let's start with the negative experiences. What made these experiences bad? Write these factors down. Now consider the most positive experiences you have had with helping professionals. What made these experiences good?

Your bad experiences may have included extremely negative behaviors, such as rudeness, ineptitude, neglect, and even malpractice. Negative experiences may have been marked by practitioners who seemed bored, uninterested in you or your experience, uncaring, and even distrustful. Perhaps you were left waiting an unreasonably long time, ignored, or spoken to rudely. Your negative experiences may have included a disorganized, dull, or dirty environment.

Did your bad-experience practitioners recommend treatment? If so, how was this explained? When told to follow recommendations, we like to understand why. We like to know what benefits to expect and to believe that the treatment will be worth our time, money, and effort (Salmon, Santorelli, and Kabat-Zinn 1998). I hope you didn't see much of yourself or your work reflected in these negative examples!

Now consider the positive examples. Positive interactions are characterized by a sense of caring, respect, good communication, and professional behavior on the part of the practitioner. Clients or patients believe that their concerns are taken seriously and that the practitioner is highly qualified, knowledgeable, and helpful. If these positive practitioners recommend treatment, you understand the reasons for their recommendations, what

Characteristics of Positive Provider–Client Experiences

Environment
- The facility is neat and clean.
- The office and staff have a well-organized appearance.

Appearance of Provider
- The provider wears professional attire.
- The provider's appearance is neat and clean.
- The provider is friendly and interested in you, and he has time for you.
- The provider has a warm, positive attitude.
- The provider makes a positive first impression.

Interactions With Provider
- You have confidence in the provider's qualifications, training, experience, and skills.
- You have enough time to express your concerns.
- The provider listens carefully and tries to understand your concerns.
- You believe the provider is genuinely interested in you and what you have to say.
- You perceive an unconditional positive regard from the provider.
- You believe that the provider respects you and your opinions.
- You trust that the provider will maintain your confidentiality and has your best interests at heart.
- If the provider recommends treatment, instructions are clearly explained and your questions are answered.

will be involved in following them, what benefits are likely to result, and what to do when you have questions. The environment is usually clean and organized.

Now think about any job you have held. In every workplace you will find people who try to do their best and others who just show up. Maybe you have even observed these contrasting behaviors at your fitness center. Have you seen personal trainers who stand around looking bored while their clients work out? Weight room monitors with their noses buried in magazines? Group exercise instructors who haven't changed their music or routine in months and who don't know their students' names? On the other hand, some of your coworkers may always look energetic and interested in their work and have smiles for everyone. Imagine you are a client in your facility. What would your impressions be? How do you think your clients see you?

No discussion of professionalism would be complete without considering professional ethics. Ethics are moral judgments of right and wrong. Professional organizations often write codes of ethics to guide the behavior of their members. A code of ethics helps to protect consumers from fraud and other unethical practices, and it helps to preserve the integrity of the profession. Fitness professionals may find that the organization through which they are certified has a code of ethics. For example, the American College of Sports Medicine (ACSM) has a code of ethics for its members (ACSM 2002; Hilgenkamp 1998). The ACSM code of ethics states that members are expected to do the following:

- Work continuously to improve their professional knowledge and skills
- Maintain high professional standards of behavior
- Protect the public from unethical conduct
- Contribute to the improvement of people's health and well-being

Your ethical conduct protects the safety and health of your clients and establishes you as a professional. For example, when you find that clients need advice or assistance outside your areas of qualification or expertise, or what is called scope of practice, you must refer these clients to physicians, counselors, or whichever professional is best suited for the situation. Admitting you cannot do it all is not a sign of weakness or limitation, but simply an acknowledgment of the scope of your training. Your clients will respect you for referring them and appreciate your concern for their well-being.

Scope of Practice

When fitness professionals give exercise advice they must be sure that they are qualified to deal with a given client's needs and that the advice they give will not lead to injury or other health problems. When you give advice regarding health issues you have not been trained or certified to deal with, you may be guilty of the unauthorized practice of medicine, which could result in legal as well as ethical problems. To be sure you stay within your scope of practice, follow these guidelines:

1. Do not diagnose health problems. Leave the diagnosis to a health professional. Even though symptoms that clients share with you may suggest a certain illness, you are not qualified to deliver a diagnosis. Instead, if the symptoms concern you, suggest that clients make an appointment to speak with a physician.

2. Ask clients to obtain medical clearance when necessary. Your employer or certifying agency should have guidelines to help you decide who needs medical clearance. If in doubt, request medical clearance. Be sure you have your clients' medical clearance before you proceed with fitness testing or exercise prescription.

3. Recommend exercise to improve health and fitness, but not to treat a medical condition. This is a technicality. We all know that exercise is great medicine and is prescribed to help treat many medical conditions. Physical activity may reduce hypertension, improve blood sugar regulation, and strengthen weak muscles. But unless you are also a health care provider, you do not have a license to provide treatment. The health care provider prescribes treatment; you work within her recommendations to design a safe exercise program.

4. Do not work with clients whose medical needs exceed your level of training. This is obvious! The last thing you want is to hurt someone. Exercise can cause injury, so err on the side of caution. Refer clients with medical needs to someone qualified to address those needs.

5. Do not provide psychological counseling when clients want to discuss personal problems. Refer them to a qualified professional. By all means, listen and express your sympathy and support, but do not offer advice or take on a counseling role.

(continued)

(continued)

6. Limit your nutrition advice to mainstream recommendations. These include using the United States Department of Agriculture Food Guide Pyramid and telling people to eat plenty of fruits and vegetables, limit empty-calorie snacks, drink plenty of water, and so forth. Refer clients who want more personalized advice to a physician or qualified dietitian. Never recommend over-the-counter supplements; few have been tested for long-term effectiveness and safety.

7. Always give sound and safe exercise advice. Your clients' health and safety are your top priorities. Stay current on exercise safety issues, and never recommend exercises that could cause harm. You may think that this advice is too conservative, but if you find yourself with an injured client in a court of law, you will be happy that you stuck with a conservative approach.

What *can* you do? In general, personal trainers and other fitness professionals are qualified to assess fitness, educate clients about safe and effective exercise, design exercise programs, and motivate and train their clients.

Maintaining the confidentiality of your clients or patients is one of your most important ethical responsibilities. Clients will often share important personal information with you, such as the health issues they face. Keep these confidences to yourself. If you wish to discuss a client's health issue with another person, ask your client's permission before doing so. For example, you may want to check with someone about the advisability of certain exercise stations for a client who has a back problem. Before calling the client's physical therapist or discussing the situation with someone else, tell your client whom you wish to contact and why. And most important, never talk about one client to another. This will cause all of your clients to wonder whether they will be the next object of discussion.

Another important ethical issue for fitness professionals is conflict of interest, which occurs when you perform one role that may negatively influence your performance of another. For example, if you were to sell supplements, it would be a conflict of interest for you to perform nutrition counseling. You might act in your own self-interest (sell as many supplements as possible) rather than in the client's best interest (recommend only appropriate supplements). A commitment to professional and ethical conduct, combined with a deep abiding respect for your clients, will help you make good decisions in your professional life.

Importance of Effective Communication Skills

By now you have a good idea of what a positive and professional provider–client relationship looks like. But how do you forge these relationships?

Begin by thinking about your clients or patients. Who are they? What are they like? If your clients or patients are similar to you, then answering these questions is easy. But if they differ from you in age, ethnicity, gender, socioeconomic status, or educational background, connecting may take research. If you find significant cultural differences between you and your clients, try to learn about their beliefs, attitudes, and lifestyles. Talk to others who work with this population. And most of all, spend time with your clients or patients and listen to what they have to say. Your advice will be more relevant, meaningful, and practical if you understand the people with whom you work.

Here's an example of the communication difficulties that can arise when fitness professionals are unfamiliar with their clients' backgrounds. A woman in her 70s was referred to a fitness center to perform resistance training to strengthen her muscles. She attended regularly and made steady progress. She appreciated the fitness center's professional staff and found them to be knowledgeable and helpful. However, one young man, a student intern from the local college who monitored the weight room occasionally, made what she found to be awkward comments. For example, in an effort to be friendly and to make conversation, at the end of the week he sometimes asked her what she was doing that weekend. When she replied, "Well, the usual," he would say, "Make your husband take you out!" The woman's husband had a disability and found leaving the house stressful. The couple enjoyed their time alone at home. Because both were retired, the weekend was no different from weekdays. As the young man became more familiar with this woman's background, his ability to converse with her improved.

The fitness industry is all about working with people. Your effectiveness depends on your ability to communicate well with people. You must be able to communicate not only with your clients, patients, or students but also with colleagues in your organization and in your community.

As health and fitness professionals we get paid to give good advice; therefore, we tend to think that the more we talk, the better our performance. We love to talk about exercise and health, and we are eager to demonstrate our expertise and knowledge. Unfortunately, our enthusiasm can get in the way of our work when we dominate conversations and interrupt speakers with our recommendations.

When we think about communication skills, we usually think about improving our ability to deliver a convincing argument and to get others to agree with us. We may think about impressing others with our wit and wisdom and our entertaining jokes and stories. But to increase our effectiveness as fitness professionals, the most important communication skill we can improve is our ability to listen. Think back to your analysis of good provider–client relationships. Which was a more important characteristic of good providers: the ability to speak eloquently or the ability to listen and understand you? Although it is important to be able to explain things clearly, your explanations will fall on deaf ears unless you have gained your clients' attention by listening carefully to their needs.

Those who work with people need to be good listeners. If you are a personal trainer or exercise instructor, you need to listen carefully to your clients to understand what concerns them and what they are looking for. Listening carefully allows you not only to receive information but also to interpret reactions to your suggestions. Listening to coworkers and clients helps you to respond most effectively to their concerns.

Our lives are so busy and noisy, we become used to tuning people out or to listening with half an ear while we think about other things. As people talk to you during the day, become aware of how much of the time you really listen. Chances are that most of the time your mind is elsewhere.

Some of the time we pretend to listen, but we don't really pay attention. We pretend to listen so that people will like us or not think us rude. We may hear only part of what the speaker says and tune out parts we find boring or offensive, or we tune out parts we don't understand. We might formulate arguments, form judgments about the speaker, or think about what we will say next. We may simply daydream about something else entirely. We might be preoccupied with ourselves, perhaps distracted by our own problems.

Even if we try to listen, we may not hear what the speaker says. We often reconstruct messages to reflect our own beliefs and needs. We may have prejudices about the speaker and look for confirmation of these in their words. We may have hidden agendas and hear only what we expect to hear.

An important listening technique you should consider using is empathetic listening, which is listening with full awareness and an open mind, trying to put yourself in the speaker's shoes. Empathetic listening is essential when a conversation is important, such as when trying to help clients design exercise programs. Listening carefully allows you to gather the information you need to successfully work with your clients and to give your clients the impression that what they say is important.

When it is time to listen carefully, make a decision to do so. Set the stage and shift your mind into listening mode. Conduct interviews with clients in a quiet and private space, and turn off the music to limit distractions. Give clients your full attention, and concentrate on what they say. You will probably ask them several questions; give them enough time to answer each one before moving on.

Show that you are listening. Make appropriate eye contact, lean forward, and take notes as necessary (but don't spend all your time writing). Ask for explanations of points you do not understand. To check your understanding, paraphrase what the speaker has said. Paraphrase emotions as well as content: "That must have been difficult." Ask open-ended questions to get more information about important topics: "You said you quit exercising last year. What made you stop?"

You can use self-disclosure to show that you understand what your client is saying. Admitting your own mistakes and problems can help you connect with others. But limit yourself to one or two sentences. Remember, the focus is on the client, not on you.

Q&A

Q What if a client shares something that worries you?

A When you are a good listener, clients may confide in you and disclose information that worries you. They may want to talk about inappropriately personal topics that make you uncomfortable. Let them know that you aren't willing to discuss these things and steer the conversation back into the fitness arena. Sometimes clients give you clues that they have serious psychological or other health problems that are beyond your professional expertise. Be sure to suggest strongly that they get professional help and let them know you are not the one to treat their alcoholism, depression, eating disorder, or whatever else may surface during your work with them. If their problems are beyond your scope of practice, you may be unable to continue working with them.

Your ability to be an effective listener and to connect with your clients or patients is one of your most important professional skills. On the surface people come to you for exercise advice. But they may also look to you for approval. They may come because they are in pain, face physical problems, or worry about health problems. In addition, many look for community and connection, even meaning, in their exercise experiences. You should not strive to become your clients' or patients' therapist or best friend, but you can acknowledge them, make a connection, and treat them with dignity and respect.

Q&A

Q What about clients who talk too much?

A Listening with your full attention takes a lot of energy, so choose when you will listen carefully. You should certainly listen mindfully when you first meet with a new client and are gathering information concerning health risks, fitness goals, and exercise program design. But do you need to keep listening with full concentration every minute you are with clients, especially clients you work with regularly and have known a long time? This depends on the relationship and is up to you. Clients or patients may stay with you because they value your ability to listen. But perhaps you have clients who drive you crazy by chattering away the entire time you are together. You may choose to listen with half an ear some of the time, tuning in when important topics come up.

When it is your turn to talk, encourage clients to paraphrase what you have told them in order to check their understanding. Pause frequently to see if they have questions. When giving advice, write everything down; people are likely to forget some of your spoken instructions. Use readable and attractive handouts to reinforce your main points. Speak slowly and clearly, and avoid unnecessary jargon.

Limit the amount of advice you deliver in a given session. As you get to know your clients or patients, you will learn how much information they want. Some are full of questions and seem ready to enroll in an exercise physiology course. They love getting a million handouts and can handle quite a bit of information. Others may become overwhelmed with too much information. Give them a few important pieces of information at a time, and keep instructions as simple as possible.

Your communication skills reflect your basic philosophy, whether philosophy creeps into your discussions or not. Your clients will sense your attitude toward them, so do your best to cultivate a respectful and understanding demeanor. Use positive, but honest, comments and observations to reinforce their strengths and enhance their self-confidence. This builds the productive working alliance that is most likely to lead to fitness success.

Self-Renewal, Stress Management, and Avoiding Burnout

Connecting with clients takes energy, so it is important to structure your work in ways that give you energy, and to create a lifestyle that nourishes your creative spirit. Each day must provide opportunities for self-renewal and stress reduction. By cultivating a stress-resistant lifestyle you can avoid the burnout that commonly occurs in the helping professions.

Your first line of defense against burnout may be your job. Although this might sound contradictory, people who create meaning in their work are more resistant to the negative health effects of stress (Ardell 1996). Believe in the importance of your work. Everything you do and say can make a difference in someone's life. Even difficult clients may have something to teach you. Use the visualizations of lifetime goals presented earlier in this chapter, in the section "Exercise Adherence and Career Development." As you strive to develop your career according to your most important goals and values, your work will become more rewarding and personally meaningful to you.

Take advantage of opportunities for professional development and continuing education. Your certifications probably require you to take classes and attend workshops and professional conferences. These experiences are tremendously rewarding. Networking with other fitness professionals provides new ideas and support for the difficulties we all face in our work and in our lives. Join a professional organization that offers conferences that address topics you find useful and interesting. And never stop reading.

Even the most interesting and rewarding work must exist in balance with our personal lives. Set strict limits on your time at work. This can be especially difficult in the fitness business, where many clients exercise outside of their workday. Classes and personal training sessions often fall during the early morning, late evening, and weekend hours. If you are not vigilant, you may find yourself working all three! Try to develop a reasonable schedule that accommodates your own needs as well as those of your family, if you have one. For example, you may decide to work late afternoons and evenings, but not early mornings or weekends.

Set boundaries so that your work does not overwhelm your personal life. Think carefully about how you would like clients to contact you. Give out your phone number only if you can turn off your phone and route calls to your voice mail. Maintain a professional distance with clients; they will respect you for this. There is no need to be on call every minute of the day. Be especially firm if you run into needy clients who try to insist you adapt to their schedules at the expense of your own.

Jobs with a mixture of teaching and administrative work provide a good variety for most fitness professionals. Because teaching and personal training take a great deal of energy, you are in danger of burnout if you have too many intense contact hours each day. Some find that work as a personal trainer or exercise instructor is a fun second job that balances their other more sedentary job. Over time you will be able to figure out what works best for you.

As you search for balance in your work, do what you can to cultivate balance in other areas of your life. Get enough rest, eat well, spend time with family and friends, and of course, engage in regular physical activity. If you are not able to find enough time for exercise, you know something is wrong! Practice what you preach.

As you devise strategies to increase exercise adherence in your work, remember that clients drop out of exercise programs for many reasons. You do not, and would never want to, control their lives. Don't take client dropout personally. Just do your best, then let go of expectations. Focus on the process, not the product.

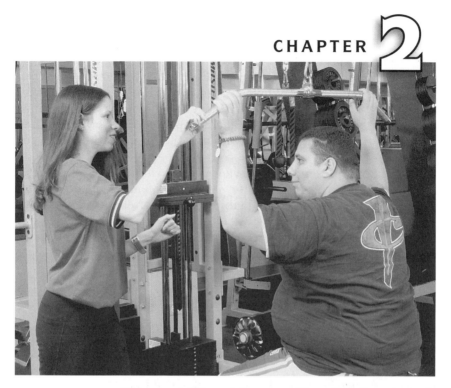

How Do People Change?

People *can* change. You have seen it happen. You have seen people change the way they think about their lifestyles. You have seen them change their attitudes toward physical activity and their feelings about their ability to become more active. You have seen clients or patients change from couch potatoes into regular exercisers. Sometimes the changes are dramatic. Perhaps you have known clients who have drastically changed their lives, maybe working fewer hours or moving to a new location, becoming more active in the process. Other times the changes are small, but they yield important health benefits. Perhaps a client or patient who is somewhat active adds resistance training to her schedule.

You have also seen people who found change very difficult, even impossible. You have seen clients try and then fail to add even small amounts of activity to their lives. One day they say they are committed to getting more exercise, but a few weeks later they quit. You may wonder what they are thinking and what their lives are like. Why do some people expend great effort to change their lives, and others change the subject when you mention a short walk?

Welcome to the world of psychology! Psychologists study the thoughts, emotions, and behaviors of humans. Much of the research on behavior change comes from the field of psychology. Psychologists have identified many factors that help us understand how people form the intention to change, initiate changes in behavior, and then sustain these changes over the years.

This chapter presents an overview of the behavior change process. Even though no two people are the same, we can make generalizations about the process that people go through when attempting to begin an exercise program. Discovering where in this process your client is can help you make more effective recommendations. This chapter also presents ideas on assessing a person's readiness for exercise.

Behavior Change Process

Unless we perceive a very good reason for changing, change goes against our nature (Vohs and Heatherton 2000). We strive for stability in order to grow and thrive. Stability, or the force of habit in our daily routine, frees us to be creative in our work and to think about things more important than self-care and the tasks of daily living. We strive, consciously and subconsciously, to maintain stability in our lives.

Behavior change usually begins when we perceive a problem or need for change. At first we may focus on the difficulty of making the change, and for a while the cons (reasons for not changing) may outweigh the pros (reasons for changing). However, we may continue to consider the idea of change. If the problem persists, we may decide that we should take action. The pros start to outweigh the cons, and we start devising schemes for making a change. We may talk to a friend about our plans and even set a date for changing behavior. We may decide to quit smoking on our birthday or start exercising when a new session begins at the local fitness center. Forming these preliminary plans helps us feel better.

Behavior change is successful when our plans come to fruition: We actually quit smoking or join the exercise class. Many factors support us during this period of behavior change. Support from our smoking cessation group strengthens our resolve. Compliments from friends and having more energy during the day enhance our perception of exercise benefits. If many of our friends and acquaintances exercise, we're more likely to stick to our exercise program. This support helps us cope with the difficulties we invariably encounter from day to day.

As time goes by, the changes we have made may become routine, and we establish a new version of stability. The force of habit helps us stay away from cigarettes or get to the gym for our workout. Our new behavior becomes more automatic, requiring less thought or self-control.

Of course, in real life, behavior change doesn't resemble a process until after we've changed our behavior and then looked back to see how we got there. Attempts to change behavior take on new shapes along the way. Even with successful behavior change we see that behavior may change again at any time, and we might resume smoking or become too busy to exercise. Or we may exercise more than we used to, but not as much as planned. At any point in the behavior change process we may move backward rather than forward. We may decide that the cost of changing our behavior is too high after all. Our plans were not realistic, our expectations too high. But we learn from our behavior change experiences, whether or not they lead to long-term success, and we use this information in our next attempt.

Most psychologists believe it is useful to think about behavior change as a process (Weinstein, Rothman, and Sutton 1998). Some psychologists view behavior change as a continuum—from no thought of changing to recognizing a need to change and then finally to taking action. Some psychologists believe it is helpful to view the process of behavior change as a series of steps, referred to as stages of change.

Stages of Change Model for Physical Activity

One of the most widely used models when thinking about changing physical activity level is the stages of change model (Prochaska, Johnson, and Lee 1998; Marcus et al. 1998). Although this model was originally used to describe attempts to quit smoking, it has been applied with success to other types of health behavior, including exercise (Marcus and Forsyth 2003; Reed 1999).

A model is only as useful as its applications. Fitness professionals have found the stages of change model helpful when working with clients to change patterns of physical activity (Marcus et al. 1998). It makes sense that you would approach a client already convinced of the benefits of physical activity very differently from the way you would talk to someone who does not recognize the value of regular exercise and has no intention of becoming more active. You probably do this already. Tailoring your actions and recommendations to a client's readiness to change can help you make the most of your time and energy.

The following are descriptions of Prochaska's (1998) stages of change, with suggestions for tailoring your exercise recommendations to meet the needs of people in each of these stages (Marcus et al. 1998; Marcus and Simkin 1994; Prochaska and Marcus 1994; Reed 1999; Riebe and Nigg 1998).

Stage 1: Precontemplation

People in this stage have no intention of changing. They do not exercise and don't intend to start. They may be unaware that their habits are problematic, or they may feel that although this behavior (such as a sedentary lifestyle) is a problem, they can't change. They may deny the extent or seriousness of the problem and use defensive strategies when others try to point out that the behavior might be a problem.

Researchers have further categorized people in this stage into non-believers and believers (Reed 1999). Precontemplation nonbelievers do not believe in the value of the change in question, that a need for change exists, or that they have the physical ability to become more active. Many remain unaware that inactivity is a serious risk factor for chronic illness. They may have no idea that a sedentary lifestyle increases the risk of heart disease, high blood pressure, type 2 diabetes, and colon cancer. They may think that people who exercise are strange and may have misunderstandings about the effects of physical activity. For example, some people who appear relatively lean believe that they don't need to exercise because exercise is only for those who need to lose weight. Some thin people even believe that exercise might make them lose more weight and become too thin. Similarly, many people experience fatigue during the day and fear that exercise will increase this fatigue; they don't realize that an appropriate level of activity increases daily energy levels. Some precontemplation nonbelievers may believe in the benefits of exercise, but may not believe that they are physically capable of exercising.

Precontemplation believers accept, at least somewhat, that physical activity is valuable, but the idea of becoming more active is just not on the radar screen. They may have read about exercise benefits or heard stories on the news. But they have not made the leap and applied this knowledge to their own lives. They do not believe that they can become exercisers. Concepts that reinforce their sedentary lifestyle are stronger than concepts of exercise benefits. Precontemplation believers may think that it takes great quantities and intensities of exercise to achieve beneficial results, quantities and intensities that are beyond their abilities. Or they may think that only sports count as exercise and have no access to organized sports. Exercise may not be valued by their culture. They may see exercise as something only other people do. Beliefs about an active lifestyle may be at odds with the beliefs people hold about themselves or their group: "It's dangerous for people my age to exercise," or "I could never wear one of those outfits."

What can you do to help those in the precontemplation stage? Many fitness professionals, such as personal trainers and exercise instructors, whose clients come to them rarely see people in the precontemplation phase. However, those working in clinical settings, public health, worksite fitness, and community-based programs with outreach components will be more familiar with this group. Precontemplators can be challenging to work with if the goal is behavior change, but these are the folks who need you the most. Many do not value what you do, and some may even think you are crazy!

Your best strategy with precontemplators, both nonbelievers and believers, is education. Even though you cannot make them form the intention to become more active, you can give them information that might help them form this intention on their own. Attractive, easy-to-read handouts containing information about physical activity are useful in many settings (Brehm 2000a). Be sure the material is at an appropriate reading level for your group. If possible, talk to your precontemplators, either individually or in groups, to find out what they think about exercise. Use your listening skills to try to understand them. Do what you can to correct misinformation, which abounds when it comes to exercise. Most people need to learn more about the dangers of a sedentary lifestyle and to broaden their concepts of physical activity.

Success Story
Resistance (to) Training

Louis was a personal trainer at a large successful fitness center. A long-term client bought her mother, Helen, five personal training sessions with Louis. She asked Louis to start her mother, age 72, on a weight training program to help her mother maintain her bone density. At their first meeting, Louis resisted the temptation to hand Helen a weight training program and give her an orientation to the weight room. Instead, he let Helen do the talking, and he discovered that Helen had no intention of exercising and that she was only meeting with Louis to appease her daughter. He discovered that Helen considered exercise a waste of time and that she knew very little about the potential benefits of exercise for older adults. Louis realized Helen was in the precontemplation stage and focused his sessions on conversation and education. At the end of her five sessions with Louis, Helen was finally convinced that regular exercise could help her, but weight training was out of the question for the time being. Helen joined a water exercise class for seniors that met two mornings a week. The water exercise helped her arthritis and improved her stamina and range of motion. After several months Helen eventually started strength training at home, using the exercises Louis suggested when she refused to go into the weight room.

Stage 2: Contemplation

People in this stage are sedentary but thinking about becoming more active. They are aware of some of the costs and benefits of becoming more active, although many misconceptions about exercise may still be present. Many adult contemplators have had exercise experiences, both positive and negative, and these influence current thoughts for better or for worse. Others may never have tried to exercise regularly. Contemplators are still weighing the pros and cons and thinking about whether to exercise regularly. They may be wondering how to begin.

What can you do to help contemplators? Like precontemplators, contemplators need information. If you are lucky enough to work with a contemplator one-on-one, as in a personal training situation, you can have a great deal of influence. If you ask good questions and listen carefully, you can find out what your clients see as the pros and cons of exercise. You can correct erroneous beliefs (exercise can help you lose 30 pounds in 30 days) and supplement the pros with motivational but correct information (exercise along with sensible eating habits will help you lose weight slowly and gradually, but the weight will stay off and you'll be healthier). You can discuss ways to deal with the cons and help clients develop exercise programs that will lead to long-term adherence. With their willingness and your guidance, contemplators can move fairly quickly to the preparation and action stages of behavior change.

If your work situation does not allow one-on-one work with contemplators, you may be able to reach small groups by holding informational and motivational talks at convenient times and places. For example, some worksite fitness programs hold informal lecture or discussion groups during the lunch hour. You are likely to attract contemplators (along with people in the next stage, preparation) with topics such as "How do I begin an exercise program?" To enhance their motivation to become more active, contemplators also want to learn more about the risks of a sedentary lifestyle and the benefits of exercise. Discussion groups can be especially motivational if members describe fitness successes, past or current. Hearing from people similar to themselves (not just you, the buff, tough super-jock they cannot relate to) enhances feelings of self-efficacy and leads your audience to thinking, *I can do this, too.*

Success Story
Warming Up to Exercise

Georgia leads a weight control group at a large community center. A firm believer in the importance of regular physical activity, she finds that many in her group focus all their weight loss efforts on their eating behavior and are fairly inactive. Intellectually they understand the importance of exercising to maintain weight loss, but they are reluctant to begin a program of regular physical activity. Many fit the contemplator profile: They think they will begin exercising sometime, but they haven't figured out how or when.

Rather than rushing into action, Georgia knows these members need time to mentally warm up to the idea of regular exercise before they can move to the preparation phase. She provides lots of information on the benefits of exercise and leads discussions on how to fit more activity into their lives. She invites group members who are exercising to talk about how they do it. After several of these sessions she invites members of her group to participate in an exercise program at her community center. Members must accumulate 50 miles of walking over six weeks to earn a free T-shirt. Many join and make plans to walk together. Georgia meets one group at the community center after work each day and gives them walking routes. In this gradual and gentle way, she moves her contemplators through preparation and into action.

Stages of Change Model: How Do You Spell Success?

Many health and fitness professionals appreciate the fact that the stages of change model implies value in helping clients move on to the next behavior change stage, even when no changes in behavior are evident. Although the best success is getting people to adopt a regular exercise habit, we must recognize that change, especially a big change like working physical activity into daily life, takes time. Sometimes we may not see change taking place in our clients. Many attempt to change, but for some reason they quit exercising, and we may never see them again. Instead of calling this a failure, we can call it a learning experience.

We never know what goes on in another person's head. Positive changes may have occurred, even for clients who dropped out of our programs. For example, they may have acquired a greater understanding of the benefits of physical activity that, in the future, will help them change from contemplation to preparation and then to action. Or perhaps one of our workshops helped precontemplators begin considering the benefits of exercise and become contemplators. An individual life is a large and complicated thing, and even though we try to exert our helpful influence, clients may not always do as we advise. We must remember to appreciate even small changes and know that our work is often helpful, even if change is not always apparent.

Stage 3: Preparation

People in this stage have decided to add more exercise to their lives and are getting ready to begin. They may have signed up for an exercise class, bought new walking shoes, or joined a health club. They may have set a start date for their first exercise session or started exercising sporadically, perhaps walking occasionally. At this point, people are believers in the health benefits of exercise, but may have many unrealistic expectations for the changes they hope to achieve by becoming more active. The exercise programs they plan may be overly ambitious. They may underestimate the time and energy their exercise plans will take and the difficulties that may arise in daily life.

People in the preparation stage are an easy mark for health club membership sales, but they are at high risk of disappointment and early dropout. Many unscrupulous individuals and organizations take advantage of the naive beginning exerciser at this stage of the game. Preparation folks are ready to begin to exercise or to lose weight and may fall prey to quick and easy schemes. The more unrealistic their expectations, the greater their future disappointment.

What can you do to help people in the preparation stage? In one-on-one personal training situations and in group sessions, you can help preparers clarify goals and expectations. Your goal is to help clients maintain their beliefs in the importance of exercise without promising them a winning lottery ticket. Regular exercise has so much to offer in the way of promoting long-term health, preventing chronic disease, and improving daily quality of life that we really shouldn't need to inflate these benefits. Unfortunately, we are competing with the "quick and easy" crooks who profit quickly and easily by making false claims about their products. As scientists and professionals we must educate our clients (and the public at large) about the actual benefits of exercise and about the misleading claims unscrupulous companies and individuals make.

Once goals are clarified, do your best to help patients and clients design exercise programs that will work best for them. As always, consider your clients' schedules, preferences, and health concerns so that they will be likely to find satisfaction in their exercise experiences. Ask those with previous exercise experience what worked best and what didn't work well. Avoid recommending exercise that could lead to discomfort or injury. Help clients build social support. Give advice on time management. And continue to educate about the importance of regular physical activity.

How do you attract people in the preparation stage? Preparers may solicit the advice of a personal trainer, but you may need to advertise so they know how to contact you. Worksite or community lecture and discussion groups can provide a good educational vehicle to help those in the preparation stage get moving. You might attract these people at an open house for your facility, especially if you promote the event as an opportunity for those new to exercise to get started. Consider letting several people similar to your audience talk briefly about their own exercise benefits and about how they became regular exercisers.

Q&A

Q Regular exercise has many health benefits, yet I sometimes feel I am promising potential clients too much. I mean, the client I am talking to may still go on to have a heart attack. And I don't really know how much weight another client can realistically lose. On the other hand, people seem to find my enthusiasm about exercise benefits motivational. If they get people moving, can these promises be too bad?

A You can show your enthusiasm and promote the benefits of exercise in a general way without making promises. For example, we know that regular aerobic exercise reduces the risk of heart attack, but you are right: Some people who exercise will still suffer a heart attack. Studies can only give us "in the long run, on the average" kinds of information. Keep your statements general. Tell your clients that exercise can help reduce a person's risk of developing hypertension, heart disease, and diabetes. This is true. If these disorders develop, or already exist, exercise can reduce their severity. Give clients interested in weight control a general range of weight losses you have seen for similar clients, while letting them know their results may vary. In this way, you do not make promises to any given individual.

Stage 4: Action

Here we go! People in the action phase are doing it. They have started to exercise, but have not yet maintained their behavior for six months. Researchers believe that the first six months of an exercise program are the most difficult (Prochaska, Johnson, and Lee 1998). People in this stage may struggle to stick to their plans. Health and fitness professionals are well acquainted with the diversity in this group. These are the people you see in your classes and facility. Some will become regular exercisers, and others will drop out over the next six months.

Some researchers (Reed 1999) believe it is helpful to break this group into two groups: action/ambivalent and action. These groups differ in confidence in their ability to become regular exercisers. People in the action/ambivalent group exercise regularly, but resemble those in the preparation group in many ways. They still search for information on structuring and sticking to their exercise programs. While the benefits of exercise, or pros, are important to them, they still grapple with the cons. Their new behavior is fragile and their likelihood of dropout is high. Their plans to exercise may be upset by day-to-day problems.

In contrast, people in the action group are more confident and are well on their way to dealing with exercise barriers. They are believers in the benefits of physical activity and in their ability to stick to an exercise program. Because people in the action stage who are new to exercise may fall out of the exercise habit, they continue to need plenty of support and reinforcement.

What can you do to help those in the action stage? Even though people in this group are exercising, treat them like people in the preparation group. Continue to educate in order to strengthen their belief in the exercise pros and weaken their belief in the cons. Personal trainers should ask clients to list their greatest barriers to exercise, then discuss ways to deal with whatever might worry them. Don't be afraid to redesign the exercise program. If the client is worried that exercise takes too much time, pare it down. Is the program too intense? Reduce target heart rate recommendations. High-intensity programs have higher dropout rates than programs of moderate intensity. Better that your clients exercise a little than not at all. Sacrifice the "perfect" program if it will help your clients stick to their exercise plans.

Ask clients to anticipate upcoming disruptions. For example, what will clients do during the holidays? When they feel tired? When the kids are sick and home from school? If clients have exercised before, what stopped them? What could they have done differently?

In group settings you can address barriers more generally. You've probably heard all the excuses by now: I don't have enough time, I'm too tired, I quit exercising over the holidays and never started again, and the dog ate my membership card. Discuss problem-solving strategies with your group or give handouts. Congratulate your action/ambivalent clients on their progress, and help them identify the exercise benefits they have achieved. Exercise benefits might be as simple as feeling relaxed after a workout, sleeping better at night, or finding that clothes fit better. Perhaps your client or patient can work with more resistance at certain strength training stations or work at a higher intensity on a cardiovascular exercise machine. Don't forget that simply showing up deserves recognition (for example, attending a certain number of exercise sessions or sticking to the program in some other way). When progress is made, hand out rewards, such as T-shirts, free classes, personal training sessions, or whatever you have at your disposal.

Q & A

Q Is there a way to predict approximately how long each stage in this model lasts? Even some kind of a range would be helpful.

A No one can say how long a person will stay in a given stage. People may stay in the same stage for a long time or move through one or two stages very quickly. They may pass through some stages many times.

As you work with clients or patients, never try to make them fit the stages of change model; that's not what it is for. Evaluate your clients' readiness to start exercise or make changes in their exercise programs. Let this insight help you plan effective interventions. Many variables affect the behavior change process, and we must never forget how complex helping people change their exercise habits can be.

Stage 5: Maintenance

People are in the maintenance stage of behavior change when they have maintained a change for six months or more. Although the new behavior is somewhat routine, many still experience constant temptation to return to their former habits, such as smoking again or exercising less (Prochaska, Johnson, and Lee 1998). Maintaining an exercise program over the course of a lifetime can be challenging, especially when you consider how much can happen during that time!

How can you help maintainers? Even though these clients or patients have maintained their exercise program a long time, don't take them or their participation for granted. They could quit at any time. Personal trainers may want to offer clients a maintenance check-in plan. At these meetings, reinforce exercise pros and discuss the progress they have made in their physical fitness and emotional health. Are clients bored? Maybe it's time for a change. Would they like to try new activities? Give suggestions tailored to their personal preferences. Would your clients like something to train for? Help them set up a periodization training schedule that peaks them for a minitriathlon, a fund-raising walk-a-thon, or whatever event you hear of or even create.

People who have reached the maintenance stage sometimes go on to become instructors or trainers themselves. Becoming an instructor can enhance the motivation to maintain the activity the person instructs. For example, people who have successfully lost weight and maintained that weight loss make great weight control program instructors. Their stories enhance the self-confidence of those attending their groups. Similarly, people who exercise regularly are great role models for those trying to establish an exercise habit. Most fitness professionals attest that preaching about exercise benefits all day is tremendously reinforcing. In addition, the environment of the fitness center supports exercise intentions. The fitness center environment, including social support and social norms, reinforces a client's attempts to maintain or improve an exercise habit.

As you think about the stages of change, remember that clients do not necessarily progress from one stage to the next. Sometimes people return to a previous stage. It's easy for clients to go from preparation back to contemplation when they perceive flaws in their plans. You have probably seen maintainers experience lifestyle disruptions that caused them to slide back to the contemplation or preparation stages. These clients or patients may plan to exercise again, but may wonder how they'll fit it in, given their new circumstances.

Assessing Stage of Change

To apply the insights from the stages of change model to your work, you must categorize your clients or patients according to approximate stage. You can do this either by asking several questions or by asking individuals to complete a brief questionnaire. Essentially, you are trying to decide which of the categories in table 2.1 best describes each person.

Table 2.1
The Five Stages of Behavior Change

Stages of change	Physical activity
Precontemplation	Not currently active, with no intention of becoming more active
Contemplation	Not currently active, but thinking about becoming more active some day
Preparation	Planning to increase physical activity level soon. Taking steps to get ready to increase activity level, or may already exercise occasionally
Action	Performing regular physical activity for less than six months
Maintenance	Performing regular physical activity for longer than six months

Adapted from Marcus et al. 1992.

Assessing Individuals

If you work with individual clients or patients, as in a personal training or physical therapy setting, talking with them is the most effective approach. Or you could prepare a simple questionnaire (see Readiness for Exercise Questionnaire for an example), but use this in conjunction with an interview. People like to talk about themselves and, given enough time, will provide more information than a questionnaire will. These conversations will allow you to connect with your clients in meaningful and motivational ways.

Readiness for Exercise Questionnaire

Check the description that best fits you.

- ☐ I do not exercise, and I do not plan to begin exercising in the next six months.
- ☐ I do not exercise, but I am thinking about starting in the next six months.
- ☐ I do not exercise, or exercise only occasionally, but I am planning to begin exercising regularly in the next month.
- ☐ I have been exercising regularly for less than six months.
- ☐ I have been exercising regularly for six months or more.

Regular exercise means three or more times a week, 20 minutes or more at a time.
[Note to health and fitness professionals: You may wish to revise the definition of regular exercise to fit your practice.
Have you guessed which stages go with each statement?
1: Precontemplation, 2: Contemplation, 3: Preparation, 4: Action, 5: Maintenance]

Adapted from Marcus et al. 1992.

As part of your first meeting with personal training clients, ask them to tell you about their current level of physical activity. Once you understand this, you will have an idea of where they belong in the stages of change model. For example, if a client is fairly active and has been so for years, you have a person in the maintenance stage. People who have been exercising somewhat regularly for two months are in the action stage. If a client tells you he is not active but has bought new shoes and just joined your tennis club, you know you are working with someone in the preparation stage.

Trainers and therapists usually see people in the later stages of behavior change, from preparation to maintenance. After all, a person who has come to you soliciting your help and advice is probably at least in the preparation stage for physical activity, if not further. Meeting with you is an example of preparation. An exception to this might be a client who was dragged in to see you, perhaps kicking and screaming, by a relative or referred by a medical professional. A person who says, "My doctor made me come see you" may not be ready to move to the action stage, but may still be in the contemplation or even precontemplation stage.

Once you have made your first attempt to categorize your clients, further questions will help you better understand them and their stages of change. The following are helpful questions for verifying your client's stage.

If You Think Your Client Is in Maintenance

Your client has been exercising regularly for at least six months. If you are just getting to know your client, you may want to ask for more information to be sure your stage assessment is accurate and to help guide future interventions.

1. What other experiences with physical activity have you had in the past? (This question will help you determine whether your client is an off-and-on lifelong exerciser.)
2. What worked best to help you stick to your exercise program?
3. What worked the least? Which factors contributed to your quitting an exercise program?

At this point, your client may have mentioned quitting in the last six months. If not, you may be able to steer the conversation in this direction.

4. During the last six months, what factors have kept you from exercising?

Of course, you would consider clients who do not exercise for two weeks because of illness, but resume once they are well, to be in the maintenance stage. On the other hand, if they are inactive more often than active, consider them to be in the action or even preparation stage, depending on their success. When clients have rarely exercised for more than a few weeks in a row, call it preparation.

5. How do you keep up your exercise program when difficulties, such as sickness, arise? Lack of time? Travel? Holidays?

People who express confidence in dealing with these disruptions and provide evidence of dealing with them effectively in the past have a good chance of continuing to do so. This confidence, combined with a regular exercise habit lasting at least six months, indicate that your clients are truly in the maintenance stage. On the other hand, people who lack confidence in their ability to stick to an exercise program and appear to be worried about exercise barriers, or cons, would profit from interventions targeting people in the action/ambivalent stage.

If You Think Your Client Is in Action

Your client has been exercising regularly, but for fewer than six months. Ask questions 1, 2, 3, and 5 on page 34. You will gather important adherence information and gain a clearer picture of the client's activity patterns.

If it looks like your client belongs in the action stage, try to determine whether the action/ambivalent profile fits. Your decision will be based on your client's confidence level expressed in the answer to question 5. Remember that those in the action/ambivalent stage lack confidence in their ability to deal with exercise barriers, and for them, the cons of exercise are nearly equal to the pros.

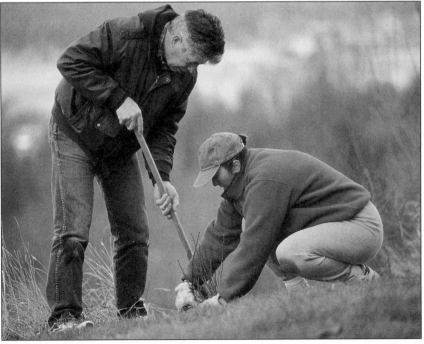

© Getty Images

Make sure your clients know that everyday activity, such as vigorous gardening, can be part of their physical activity goals.

If You Think Your Client Is in Preparation

Your client does not exercise much but is preparing to begin soon, perhaps in the next month. Some in this group are hard to peg. If they exercise a little, they may look like they belong in the action phase. Ask them questions 1, 2, and 3. If they have experience with exercise, ask question 5. If you still doubt their readiness, treat them as preparers. Bolster their confidence and help them deal with exercise barriers.

If clients appear reluctant to begin an exercise program, have had many "failures" (what we call learning experiences), and seem concerned about exercise cons, they may belong in the contemplation group. If in doubt, consider them contemplators and put a lot of energy into education. Remember, contemplators need more information about exercise benefits and about how to deal with barriers. They also need help increasing their confidence in their ability to exercise.

If You Think Your Client Is in Contemplation

Contemplators are not currently active, but thinking about becoming active, perhaps within six months. If your clients have experience with exercise, ask questions 1, 2, 3, and 5. Your job is to help them get ready to get ready for exercise (move from contemplation to preparation). Your discussions should focus on promoting the importance of exercise pros and learning how to deal with the cons.

If You Think Your Client Is in Precontemplation

People who are precontemplation believers know a little about the importance of regular physical activity, but can't see themselves adopting an exercise habit. Questions 1, 2, 3, and 5 may still provide useful information for those who have tried exercising. Some precontemplation believers have had no experience with exercise. Ask what keeps them from becoming more active. You know your clients are in the precontemplation stage when they say, "I can't exercise." Your response should be, "Why not?" Explore these issues in a supportive and tactful way. Was exercise too difficult? Do they know that exercise of moderate intensity can be comfortable and still provide many health benefits? Do they believe that exercise takes lots of time? Let them know they may begin by slightly increasing their current activity level, for example, walking only 15 or 20 minutes a day. Are they worried about the cost of joining a fitness center? Help them imagine a regular walking program they can do from home.

People who tell you they do not intend to exercise and that exercise is a waste of time are probably precontemplation nonbelievers. Ask them what they know about exercise benefits: Did you know that inactivity increases your chances of developing heart disease? Hypertension? Ask them what kind of health problems run in their families. What are their health concerns? Maybe you can link exercise to some of these. People in this stage will not consider exercising until they believe it has something to offer them.

Assessing People in a Group Setting

If you work with groups of people, with little one-on-one contact, a questionnaire is the best way to figure out how ready the people in your group are to adopt an exercise program. You may want to include the simple Readiness for Exercise Questionnaire (page 33) on forms you already use in your program, such as your medical clearance form, or as its own questionnaire.

At the bottom of the form is a short definition of *regular exercise*. If you are going to develop your own questionnaire, begin by writing your own definition. You may want to replace "regular exercise" with "regular physical activity," depending on your group. Some groups may include members who lead physically active lives performing manual labor, chasing children, climbing stairs, and so forth, but they may not think

Physical Activity or Exercise?

Physical activity refers to any type of physical movement, whereas *exercise* refers to a certain type of physical activity that is engaged in to improve physical fitness. If you walk for 20 minutes at three miles per hour to lose weight and improve your endurance, you are exercising. If you walk for 20 minutes at three miles per hour to pick up a prescription from the pharmacy, you are performing physical activity.

What's the difference between the two terms? Both offer the same beneficial effects. But the word *exercise* has a negative connotation for many. Your target population may be able to see themselves walking their errands, but not joining a health club and walking on treadmills. Because *physical activity* is a much broader term, many health and fitness professionals use it when asking people about their activity patterns. If your goal is to encourage a large group to become more active, you would promote physical activity, including housework, yard work, and transportation activities, not just exercise.

What if you work in a fitness center? Most of your clients are exercisers, and you probably are interested in promoting organized exercise that requires joining your club. Many people enjoy this option. They like the structure and organization, the supportive environment, and the fitness benefits. Of course, many of your clients may perform both exercise and other physical activities. They may enjoy your weight training class, but also walk with a friend on the weekends.

of themselves as exercising. Other groups of people are comfortable with the idea of exercise.

Your definition of regular exercise or physical activity will vary somewhat depending on your group. Many fitness professionals define adequate physical activity as exercising three to five times per week for 20 to 60 minutes per session at a fairly vigorous intensity that increases breathing rate or causes you to sweat (ACSM 1998). Activities that may reach this intensity include brisk walking, jogging, bicycling, rowing, aerobic dancing, and vigorous house and yard work. People in the public health arena may adopt the following definition: engaging in about 30 minutes of moderately vigorous activity at least five days a week (Pate et al. 1995). But these definitions may not be appropriate for an older or less able population.

What are you assessing readiness for? Joining your club? Weight training? Signing up for your group exercise class? This chapter discusses physical activity in general, but you can apply this model to a specific component. Perhaps you want to know if people in your worksite fitness program would be interested in signing up for a strength training program, or whether those signed up are likely to attend regularly. Instead of asking about regular exercise, ask about their experience with strength training. The categories on your questionnaire might resemble table 2.2.

Table 2.2

Adapted Readiness for Exercise Questionnaire (Strength Training)

Stage	Statement
Precontemplation	☐ I do not participate in strength training exercise and I do not plan to begin a strength training program in the next six months.
Contemplation	☐ I do not participate in strength training exercise, but I am thinking about starting a strength training program in the next six months.
Preparation	☐ I do not participate in strength training exercise, but I am planning to begin a strength training program in the next month.
Action	☐ I am currently performing strength training regularly, and have been training regularly for less than six months.
Maintenance	☐ I have been performing strength training regularly for six months or more.

Similar questionnaires could be prepared for a smoking cessation or weight control program.

What will this questionnaire tell you? People in the contemplation and preparation stages might be interested in a strength training program. Of course, you would need to add questions about the kind of program they might like, what times would be convenient, and so forth. Those in the action and maintenance phase may be interested in joining your program, or they may be happy exercising somewhere else.

Knowing what stage the people in your market are in can help you match them to interventions. Admitting only those in similar stages to a program, for example, people in the preparation and action stages, allows you to tailor your interventions to their needs. Setting up an exercise program for people in the contemplation stage is fruitless; they are not ready to take action. A better action would be to steer them into a more appropriate program.

Success Story
Setting the Stage

Shari uses the concept of stage-based tailoring in her worksite fitness program. One of the classes she runs is a cardiovascular risk-reduction program for those with at least one risk factor for cardiovascular disease. This eight-week program helps participants establish exercise habits and provides information about other risk factors. Of the programs in Shari's department, this is the most expensive to run, and her supervisor watches her results like a hawk. Shari needs to show her supervisor that a significant number of her previously sedentary participants still exercise six months after the program's completion. Two years ago Shari added a stages of change questionnaire to the program's application form and began admitting primarily people in the preparation and early action stages to her program. She also conducts brief presession telephone interviews with each potential participant to confirm that they are ready to start an exercise program and to share her expectations in terms of their regular participation. Shari eliminated people in the precontemplation stage who used to sign up for the program because it sounded like a good way to get a break from work and because they liked the free lunches. Her adherence figures improved greatly after she made these changes in the application process. Her supervisor is happy with the adherence data and Shari believes that her energy and the company's money are well spent on this program.

Stages of Change and Adherence

Most programs with the goal of increasing physical activity are designed for those in the preparation and action stages, people who have decided to become more active and are psychologically prepared to sign up for a class or program. They have weighed the exercise pros and cons and have convinced themselves that the pros will be worth the effort. They have thought about the complications that might arise and have worked out possible solutions. They have gathered information about exercise and are more or less ready to begin. People in the preparation and action stages sign up for exercise classes or programs, and hopefully attend them.

But what about the contemplators and precontemplators? Sometimes contemplators sign up for programs on the spur of the moment because friends signed up or a discount was tempting. But unless contemplators truly believe that exercise benefits outweigh the costs and take steps to accommodate exercise in their schedule, they may soon flounder and quit. People in the earlier stages of change need time to go through the change process. They cannot jump immediately into action.

The stages of change model suggests that programs with a variety of activities tailored to a wide range of stages should exert the greatest impact. Therefore, in addition to traditional classes and programs for those in the preparation and action stages, activities for those in the precontemplation and contemplation stages should be offered. Health fairs, lectures, handouts, and workshops promoting the benefits of exercise and educating about the dangers of a sedentary lifestyle may provide these folks the information they need to move forward.

Understanding the behavior change process can help you see your clients and your potential clients with new eyes and help you meet them with new ideas. Many fitness professionals assume that each person who comes to them is convinced of the value of regular physical activity and ready to jump into an exercise program. Avoiding a one-size-fits-all approach allows you to acknowledge the diversity in exercise-adoption readiness and meet your clients or patients where they are in the behavior change process. It encourages a client-centered approach to motivation and adherence that is most likely to bring long-term success, for you and for them.

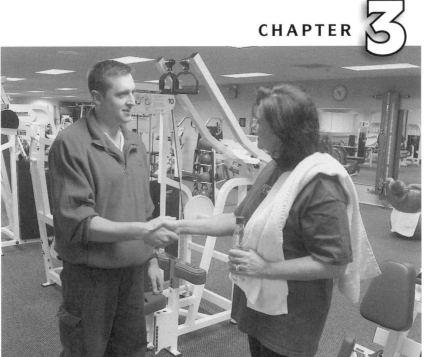

CHAPTER 3

© Jim Whitmer

Promoting Adherence From Day One

You meet with a new client for the first time. You smile, shake hands, and say thanks for being on time. Perhaps you already know quite a bit about this person based on the forms he submitted in advance. You begin by asking, "What do you hope to accomplish through an exercise program?" Once you have a general idea of your client's motivation, instead of rushing into an exercise prescription, you try to determine his readiness for regular exercise. Then you begin to formulate a plan that will enhance his motivation and adherence. Although you may be formulating an exercise program in your head, you know it will not be ideal if he quits after a few weeks.

You also know that this first meeting is the most important you will have with this client. For one thing, it may be your only meeting. For another, it sets the tone for your working relationship, if one develops, and for the work to follow. At this point you know that writing an exercise prescription is the easy part; getting your client to establish an exercise habit is the tricky part. Your goal in this first meeting is to help your client establish the foundation for a lifelong exercise habit.

Now that you are familiar with the stages of change model, you understand the range of readiness you will meet in your work. Many fitness professionals (and people in general) tend to see what they expect to see. In our case, we may expect to see people ready to exercise regularly. We may assume that our clients are eager to get started. Most clients want to make a good impression and to meet our expectations. They mean what they say when they tell you they want to take on the exercise program you help them design. But sometimes the positive image a client projects does not represent the whole story, the complicated picture of an individual juggling many responsibilities and coping with stress and changing emotional needs. Your job when meeting with a client is to try to perceive the larger picture of that client's life, so that your exercise advice will be effective.

In the previous chapter you learned how to assess your clients' readiness to engage in regular physical activity and what sort of approach to take in each stage. This chapter presents additional ways to motivate them and help them avoid common pitfalls that lead to early attrition. This information is presented in a step-by-step format. We begin with special advice for motivating precontemplators and contemplators. Next we discuss the importance of helping your clients make their health a priority and of making health concerns and fitness goals the motivational foundation for exercise program design.

This chapter also examines how to avoid common problems that lead to exercise dropout. For example, clients with unrealistic expectations are likely to become disappointed and drop out of their exercise programs. This chapter discusses how to encourage realistic goal setting despite our tendency to set unrealistic goals and overestimate our ability to stick to an exercise program.

Although your time may be limited during this first meeting with your client, you will want to take a brief look at exercise history to determine what has worked and what has created stumbling blocks. Use this information to finalize your exercise program design. Before saying good-bye to your client, help him anticipate the next step, perhaps the first day of the new exercise program, so he will be ready to start his new routine. This holistic and comprehensive approach to writing an exercise prescription will help you maximize your client's potential, which should set him up for long-term adherence and fitness success.

Step 1: Stage Your Motivational Approach

Is your client ready to take on an exercise program? After a few minutes of preliminary conversation and assessment, you are ready to steer the conversation in a direction tailored to your client's needs. Although your time at this first meeting may be limited, you use good listening and communication skills to gain enough information to guide her thinking in productive ways.

One of the issues you try to discern, using the information from the previous chapter, is whether or not your client has made the decision to stick to an exercise program. Is she convinced that the benefits outweigh the costs? Is she ready to start exercising? If so, she is either in the preparation or action stage and will benefit from your exercise advice.

On the other hand, if you find your client is skeptical of the benefits of exercise or her ability to become more active, you will waste your time and energy (and probably lose this client) if you jump right into exercise program design. You know that precontemplators and contemplators have not committed themselves mentally to becoming more active. Your work with these clients must focus on education and on exploring the ideas and barriers that prevent them from becoming more active (see figure 3.1). One of the tools for helping precontemplators and contemplators take the next step is motivational interviewing.

Q&A

Q You say it is a waste of time to design an exercise program for clients not yet ready for exercise. I occasionally see these clients, and I have doubts about their ability to stick to an exercise program. They seem tentative and unsure of themselves. But because they pay me for exercise advice, I feel obligated to write them an exercise program. Wouldn't it be wrong to send them away without at least trying to help them get started?

A By all means, write these clients the simplest, easiest-to-follow exercise program you can imagine. Who knows, maybe they will give it a try and find that they like it! But instead of spending most of your session describing how to increase the strength of the various muscle groups, spend more time helping these clients make the decision to commit to regular exercise. Go ahead and discuss health concerns and fitness goals, just as you would with any client, but keep your

(continued)

(continued)

recommendations easy to follow. Your goal is to write a program they will stick to. Adherence overrides fitness goals. Start them slowly and easily, and if they continue to exercise, you can add more exercise later. Don't be afraid of underestimating your contemplators' abilities. If they have joined a fitness facility and want to use machines, get them started on a few pieces of equipment. If they want strength training, start them with just five or six stations. If they want to exercise on their own, encourage them to walk 15 or 20 minutes a day or whatever is appropriate for their current health and fitness levels. Be sure to express confidence in their ability to follow an exercise program. Don't let your pessimism show. Bolster their self-confidence and give advice on making exercise convenient and fun.

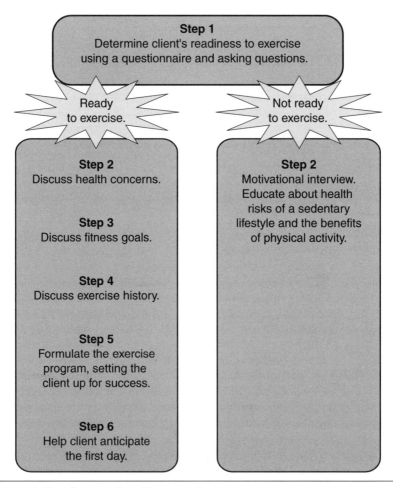

Figure 3.1 Your first meeting with a new client.

Motivational Interviewing

Motivational interviewing refers to a method of talking to people who are in the early stages of behavior change in order to direct their thinking toward a decision to increase their level of physical activity. It also shows supportive concern. Motivational interviewing was originally designed for counselors working with patients in alcohol addiction treatment programs, but the basic methods have been applied to other behavior change programs (Miller and Rolnick 1991). And even though psychologists working in addiction treatment require extensive training, health and fitness professionals with good communication skills can use motivational interviewing techniques when discussing physical activity with their patients and clients.

Your goal with inactive people is to get them to see that a sedentary lifestyle is likely to lead to future health problems. You want to help them establish two facts: Good health is important to them, and a sedentary lifestyle is dangerous to their health and well-being. Most people agree with the first statement. But you may need to convince them that their desire to be healthy requires them to become physically active.

As you talk about health and physical activity with your early-stage clients, you will be most successful if you remember the following:

- Listen carefully. Effective listening skills were reviewed in chapter 1. Listen with attention, warmth, and empathy. Even if you do not support your client's decision to remain sedentary, you must acknowledge his thoughts and feelings, and his freedom to choose. Listening carefully will show that you respect him, even if you do not condone his sedentary lifestyle.

- Educate about the dangers of a sedentary lifestyle and the health benefits of regular physical activity. Use attractive, easy-to-read handouts, and quote reliable sources. Ask questions about what you are saying to be sure your client understands the information.

- Keep the conversation friendly, and avoid argument. Negative emotions such as anger can cloud the logic you are trying to present. If you sense that your client is becoming angry or defensive, change your strategy and ask a more neutral question. Express empathy for the difficulties your client faces.

- Build self-confidence by helping clients identify areas of success. Help clients believe they can become more active if they really want to. Help them want to.

- If clients seem ready to consider the possibility of becoming more active, let them suggest ways to add activity to their lives. While at this stage clients may not be ready to leap into activity, considering the possibilities may help them move in the right direction.

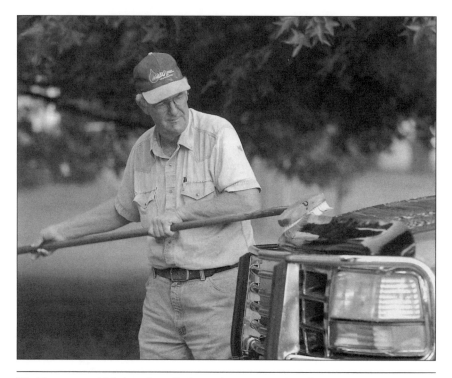

Washing your vehicle is a chore that can also count as exercise.

Begin your motivational discussion with open-ended questions that will help you and your client conclude that physical activity is important and perhaps even come up with options for increasing physical activity. Sample questions include the following (Goldstein et al. 1998; Miller and Rolnick 1991):

1. Ask about daily activity. "Tell me about your activity during a typical day. Do you walk? Do you garden?" Remember that some people do not realize that many of their daily activities count as beneficial physical exercise. Ask about housekeeping, stair climbing, and chores your client is likely to do.

2. Ask about physical activity in the past compared to now. "Has your level of activity changed over the years? What was your activity level like before you had children? Moved to this city?"

3. Briefly discuss the importance of physical activity in maintaining good health and preventing chronic disease. Then ask questions to discern how much your client knows about this. "Did you know that regular physical activity helps to prevent heart disease? High

blood pressure?" As you discuss health concerns, ask your client if he is worried about health issues, or if health problems run in his family. If health concerns relevant to physical activity come up, ask about them. For example: "Did you know that regular physical activity could help you prevent type 2 diabetes?"

4. Tell your client that you believe more activity would be beneficial and why. "I believe that regular physical activity could help you lose weight and lower your blood pressure. What do you think? Would you like more information on exercise and high blood pressure?"

5. If your client is still listening, ask about possible next steps. "You said that two years ago you enjoyed walking with friends during your lunch hour. Do you think you might like to try that again? What other activities might you be able to do?"

As you speak with a client in the precontemplation or contemplation stage, you may sense that she has stopped listening. Stop talking and encourage her to start talking again. Ask her what she is thinking about.

Should you make your clients feel somewhat uncomfortable about being sedentary? Yes. Mild discomfort may motivate them to change. After all, if you are sympathetic and reassuring, maybe they will continue to feel okay about not changing. Your job is to be supportive of them as people (*they* are okay), but to challenge their sedentary behavior (their *behavior* is not okay and could be harmful to their health).

Success Story
Outside the Comfort Zone

Evan works part time as a personal trainer in addition to his primary job as a physical therapist in a large medical center. He recently made the following observations: "It can be really discouraging to work with people who just won't commit to their exercise programs. Almost all of physical therapy involves some kind of exercise prescription, usually stretching and strengthening exercises. But many of the patients I work with have given up hope. Depression is a major problem. They are so immobilized by their physical problems, such as surgery, stroke, heart disease, and so forth, that they just can't summon the energy to exercise. Plus, sometimes the exercise is uncomfortable. I tease, I cajole, I challenge, and I bribe. Whatever will get them moving.

"That's one of the reasons I went into personal training. It's great to work with motivated people who really want my advice and appreciate

(continued)

Success Story   (continued)

my expertise. But still, sometimes I have clients who don't really want to start exercising, but their doctors have referred them to me. I have seen what can happen when health disappears. I tell them horror stories about patients I have worked with, patients who suffered heart attacks and can no longer work, patients who broke hips because their bones were frail and their muscles weak. I don't know if scaring people works, but it does seem to connect with some clients. I tell them, 'This doesn't have to happen to you if you start exercising now while you're still young and healthy.' I say, 'You want to have a heart attack? Go ahead, forget about exercise. You don't care if you live or die. You're too busy.'

"Do I worry about turning clients off, scaring them away? Not really, because I only get confrontational when I feel the client is about lost anyway. Otherwise I am enthusiastic and supportive. Some of the clients I have pushed hard are still with me, and they have told me that my challenging them forced them to confront their health issues and their sedentary lifestyle. And those I never see again? Maybe I get them thinking."

How Do Precontemplators and Contemplators Make the Decision to Change?

Information alone rarely leads to behavior change. Before people will change a behavior, they must want to change. The drive to change grows out of intellectual understanding (your information is still helpful) and emotional needs. People often decide to change when they become uncomfortable with the way things are. Psychologists have categorized some of the processes that lead to the decision to change (Courneya and Bobick 2000). The following sections describe the processes that are most relevant to fitness professionals working with clients in the precontemplation and contemplation stages of change.

Consciousness-Raising

Consciousness-raising refers to raising people's awareness of important personal issues. Clients learn about the dangers of a sedentary lifestyle in many ways, including your efforts to raise their awareness. They might receive feedback from health professionals about their personal health status. For example, a client might be diagnosed with hypertension. Or learning that certain health problems run in the family might create a desire to increase physical activity. For example, a healthy young woman may become concerned about increasing her bone density after her beloved grandmother falls and breaks a hip.

Pressure from family and friends may also raise consciousness and create discontent and motivation to change. This pressure may occur in response to perceived health problems, in which your client's family and friends believe that physical activity could help forestall a second heart attack, relieve stress, or promote weight loss. And consciousness-raising can occur through motivational interviewing as you try to help people change their attitudes about their need for physical activity.

Emotional Relief

Relief occurs when people decide to become more active and this decision eases the discomfort caused by the realization that their sedentary lifestyle jeopardizes their health. Once people experience discomfort about their lifestyles, the decision to exercise feels good and relieves stress (Pochaska and Marcus 1994). Psychologists call this process *dramatic relief.*

Chronic feelings of stress can nudge people toward lifestyle change. Events that lead people to realize they are aging or gaining weight often motivate them to begin exercise programs. Upcoming class reunions, getting together with old friends, or finding that clothes are tighter are examples. Psychologists who study behavior change use the phrase *crystallization of discontent* to refer to the discomfort that motivates people to consider adopting a new habit (Heatherton and Nichols 1994). Making the decision to exercise provides immediate emotional relief, even before the decision is acted on.

Concern for Family and Friends

Sometimes people are motivated to change because they feel their old patterns of behavior have negative effects on family and friends. For example, a mother may begin exercising because she feels tired and irritable much of the time and hopes that regular activity will relieve stress and give her more energy when she is with her family. A man who recently received a knee replacement may commit to regular exercise to regain mobility and independence so he can get back to work and support his family.

Self-Reevaluation

People confronted with the need to adopt an exercise program may experience a change in their values, a change that supports their decision to begin exercising. Health and fitness professionals often meet busy patients or clients who experience a revelation when they start to believe, *It's okay to put myself first sometimes and take care of my health.* Or people may realize that if they value their work or families, they must value their health and make time for self-care. The process of self-reevaluation can change people's self-concepts from "I can't exercise because I am too busy doing more important things" to "I must make time to exercise and take care of myself so that I can continue to do the things I need to do."

People making a decision weigh the pros and cons. What are the costs of beginning an exercise program? What are the benefits? You can help people take a good look at these factors. Remember that decisions are not based on rational thoughts alone, although rational thinking can help people make the decision to exercise. Rather, decisions are also driven by the values and emotional experiences attached to the pros and cons. Your job is to strengthen the values of the exercise pros and help people come to terms with the cons.

Step 2: Discuss Health Concerns

As you saw in the previous section of this chapter, discussing health concerns is an important focus of motivational interviews with clients in the precontemplation and contemplation stages. This is an important step in building the foundation of the exercise program. Discussing health concerns is also important when working with clients in other stages, but the discussion will focus more on exercise program design.

Most personal trainers and other fitness professionals will find that their clients are in at least the preparation or action stage and are eager for exercise advice. Once you know they are ready to start an exercise program you will want to get right to work. Skip the intense discussion of the dangers of a sedentary lifestyle for now and get right to the clients' personal health concerns and fitness goals.

What are your clients' health concerns? Health concerns serve not only as motivation to be physically active, they also provide the foundation for your exercise prescription. Health concerns may be the reason clients have contacted you in the first place. Your client has probably filled out medical forms, but ask questions aloud as well. Many clients forget to write important information on their forms, especially if they filled them out in a hurry. As you question clients about health concerns, ask not only about current concerns, but also about health problems that run in their families. As you know, exercise helps prevent, postpone, and treat many chronic health problems, such as hypertension, type 2 diabetes, and obesity (Booth and Chakravarthy 2002).

Regular physical activity has been shown to reduce symptoms of many emotional health problems, such as depression and anxiety, and to reduce feelings of stress. In fact, stress reduction is one of the primary reasons people stick to their exercise programs. For this reason, ask clients about their stress levels at this first meeting and suggest that exercise might be beneficial (Brehm 2000b).

Of course, if clients have health problems beyond the scope of your expertise, obtain medical clearance for them to work with you, or refer them to a specialist qualified to prescribe exercise for them. If you are qualified to work with them, work closely with their health care providers to ensure that your recommendations are appropriate. Take good notes about your clients' health status, and be sure to accommodate chronic injuries and health problems in your exercise prescription.

Many fitness professionals work with facilities that perform health screenings for their clients. Information about personal health risks such as blood pressure, blood sugar, blood lipids, and body fat levels can motivate clients to increase physical activity and can provide information for your exercise prescription.

Give clients information on preventing or improving the health problems that worry them. Remind them that people tend to take good health for granted until they get sick. Remind them that it is easy to postpone self-care and to become overwhelmed with their daily responsibilities. But self-care must become one of these responsibilities. Many clients have a hard time accepting the fact that regular physical activity is at least as important as everything else calling for their attention.

Step 3: Discuss Fitness Goals

After you have discussed health concerns move on to fitness goals, which will create a structure for the exercise program. What fitness improvements do clients hope to achieve? They may have shared their goals with you on paper, but discuss these and give them time to explain what they mean by vague phrases such as "better fitness" or "improved appearance." Clients may have other goals, but were too embarrassed to list them, or they may have written down things they felt they should have, such as lose 20 pounds, because they thought you would be worried about their extra fat. Do your clients have fitness test results? If so, these may help guide some of your recommendations for fitness goals.

Less experienced fitness professionals will jump right into exercise program design at this point. This is what we have been trained to do, after all! We know what is recommended for reducing blood pressure, improving muscle tone, or training for a marathon. We know which exercises will help build shoulder strength or stretch tight hamstrings. Need to lose six inches around the waist? No problem.

Or is it? Fitness professionals talk a lot about setting goals. But clients often come up with unrealistic goals, and unfortunately, fitness professionals may focus on these goals instead of on clients. In other words, if clients seek dramatic improvement in appearance and great muscle tone, a personal trainer may set them up with extremely demanding exercise programs. These exercise programs may indeed be recommended to accomplish the clients' goals, but they may not match the clients' abilities, lifestyles, time limitations, or even initial fitness levels. The result? Great exercise programs, but nobody following them.

Where Do Exercise Recommendations Come From?

Most exercise recommendations are drawn from research by exercise physiologists using information gathered in laboratory studies measuring fitness improvement in subjects undergoing various exercise training programs. These scientists focus primarily on the physical response to various forms of overload. They measure the effects of different types of training on energy production systems, blood chemistry, body composition, muscle strength, and so forth.

This valuable information helps to guide our exercise recommendations. These studies show us how much and what type of exercise can be expected to lead to improvements in cardiovascular fitness, muscle strength, and flexibility. We know the best kinds of exercise to improve blood sugar regulation and blood lipids, and to reduce high blood pressure. But as is often the case with science, it is easy to lose sight of the whole picture. The recommended amount of exercise required to achieve clients' goals may exceed the time and energy clients are willing to spend on physical activity. Our clients are not subjects in a laboratory study. As we prescribe exercise for them, we must be guided not only by the health and fitness improvements they hope to obtain, but by the other factors that influence human behavior.

Continue to use your knowledge of exercise physiology, but your first goal when working with people new to exercise and people who have trouble sticking to an exercise program for more than a few months, is to help them establish a lifelong exercise habit. Help new clients set attainable goals they can reach with a realistic exercise program.

Use your experience and expertise to guide your clients as you work together to set fitness goals. Encourage clients to be realistic. Set specific, measurable goals and record them on a page you and your clients will refer to frequently. Break down goals into small steps, steps that clients can accomplish in fairly short time periods. Suggest additional goals that are easy to meet. Many people report feeling more energetic, sleeping better, or feeling less stressed within a few weeks of beginning

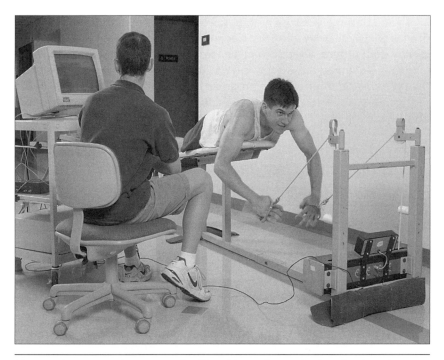

The exercise prescriptions we are familiar with are the result of studies done by exercise physiologists in human performance laboratories.

an exercise program. Encourage clients to add these to their list of goals if appropriate.

Discuss what types of exercise will help clients reach their health and fitness goals. When it is time to come up with a specific exercise plan, incorporate these activities, taking into account your clients' preferences, access to facilities, and so forth, as you always do when designing exercise programs. Be sure clients understand why the exercise program looks the way it does, and why they are doing what is planned. Help them understand the improvements they are likely to see and when they are likely to see them.

Goals for people new to exercise should focus on the *process* of exercising, not only on the *product*. For many clients, success is getting to the weight room twice a week and completing a strength training workout. Success is adding five minutes of cardiovascular exercise each session every few weeks until reaching a certain exercise duration. Success might be adding a new station to a resistance training program. Tracking workouts is a powerful motivation tool. Completing an exercise session represents the completion of a goal, when the goal is participation (Annesi 2002a).

If you continue working with a new client, reevaluate her health and fitness goals every few months. Because some clients see progress more slowly than others, your predictions for how long it would take to reach a certain goal may have been too optimistic. Let your client know that everyone is different; slower progress is not her fault, but a byproduct of the nature of statistical prediction! Revise goals when you know more about your clients.

Tips for Setting Health and Fitness Goals That Motivate Clients for Long-Term Adherence

- Listen carefully to understand what clients hope to accomplish through their exercise programs.
- Help them define measurable goals.
- Suggest additional goals they may not have thought of, such as feeling more energetic and less stressed.
- Break large goals (reachable in six months or more) into small goals (reachable in about 8 to 10 weeks) and even weekly goals, such as completing a certain number of exercise sessions.
- Include many process goals, or goals that can be reached simply by completing a workout.
- Record goals and set up a system to record workouts and track progress toward goals.
- Be sure clients understand what types of exercise will help them reach their health and fitness goals.
- Reevaluate and revise goals and exercise recommendations periodically to prevent discouragement if large goals are not met.

Great Expectations: A Double-Edged Sword

Regular physical activity yields remarkable health and fitness benefits. We spend lots of time educating our clients and potential clients about the wonderful benefits of regular exercise. And indeed, clients are sufficiently motivated by these promised benefits to come to exercise classes, join a fitness center, or work with personal trainers.

But what happens when these benefits are not immediately apparent? Sure, muscle tone will improve, but how much will the client's appearance really change? Exercise can help people lose weight, but only in conjunction with changes in eating behavior, and usually very slowly.

Think back over your experiences with all of the clients you have known. How many lost a great deal of weight? Significantly changed their physiques? How long did these changes last? What kinds of measurable benefits have your clients actually achieved? Many clients improve muscle tone and lose weight. Fitness test results may improve. Many people feel more energetic and less stressed. Some lower their blood pressure or cholesterol. These are important changes, but they may not be as dramatic as some expect.

And some clients hope for dramatic effects. Where do these great expectations come from? Some people develop an expectation for dramatic results from advertisements for products promising quick, unrealistic changes in weight or appearance. Their expectations can be reinforced by fitness professionals trying to motivate them. And some of this optimism and desire for dramatic results is part of human nature; hope does indeed spring eternal in the human breast.

The Hard Sell and Exercise Dropout

Promises, promises. Our consumer-driven culture looks for products that promise fast and easy solutions to complex problems. Wouldn't it be nice if we could find an easy way to look great and stay healthy? We hope that a product, pill, or exercise machine out there can turn back the clock on sagging muscles, or help us take off extra weight with minimal time and effort. Products that promise fast, unrealistic results create short- and long-term problems. In the short term, these products usually don't deliver as promised. In the long term, these unrealistic promises encourage the kind of thinking and beliefs that undermine healthful lifestyles. Products that promise unrealistic results lead people to believe that quick and easy is the way to go and anything that takes too much time or energy is wrong.

Some fitness professionals feel we must compete with the advertising for these products and their promises. And, of course, we can't. When competing with quick and easy solutions, exercise presents two major drawbacks: It is neither quick nor is it easy. Rather it takes time and it takes energy. Because of this, exercise can be a difficult product to sell, and we may be tempted to inflate the changes a client may expect. Attractive promises are tempting to make. You may sell a membership, sign up a personal training client, or get a new member to join your group exercise class. High expectations motivate clients to begin exercising.

But as you know, beginning an exercise program is the easy part. The hard part is staying with it. Creating unrealistic expectations ultimately results in exercise dropout. Clients eventually feel disappointed in the results (or lack of results) of their exercise programs. Some even become disappointed in themselves, feeling they have failed to work hard enough or long enough, when in reality, their goals were simply unrealistic. Clients who do not achieve their expectations are more likely to drop out of their exercise programs (Sears and Stanton 2001).

The False Hopes Syndrome and the Planning Fallacy

Even if you do not oversell the benefits of regular exercise, your clients may still develop unrealistic expectations. Your clients are human, and it is human nature to set unrealistic goals and expect unrealistic results. We may have tried and failed to lose weight 30 times before, yet we still expect our next attempt to succeed. Health psychologists call this the *false hopes syndrome* (Polivy and Herman 2000).

Why do people repeatedly start new exercise or diet programs despite past failures? Because planning and committing to these programs temporarily makes people feel better. They recognize the need for exercise, and establishing a plan makes them feel better. Their self-image immediately improves. Beginning an exercise program induces feelings of optimism and control. But then many people become overconfident in their ability to carry out their self-improvement schemes. As researchers in this area of psychology have observed (Polivy and Herman 2000, 128), "Overconfidence breeds false hope, which engenders inflated expectations of success and eventually the misery of defeat."

The *planning fallacy* is similar in nature. Psychologists have observed that whether we plan to lose weight or plan to build a space shuttle, we consistently underestimate the time, money, and energy required to accomplish our goals (Buehler, Griffin, and Ross 1994). You may have observed that construction projects almost always take longer and cost more than original projections. On a smaller scale, starting a new program at work usually takes longer to design and implement, and may cost more than originally thought. What about an exercise program? A plan that looks great on paper turns out to take much more time and energy than we have at our disposal.

Understanding this human tendency to think big can help you help your clients as you work together to come up with reasonable and successful exercise programs. Encourage them to think about past experiences with exercise programs, and nudge them in the direction of realistic aspirations. By all means nurture their hope and optimism that they can stick to their exercise plans. But use it to build an exercise program that will lead to feelings of success.

Success Story

Reality Check

Allison is a personal trainer at a large fitness center and has found that people of all ages are likely to overestimate how much time they can realistically commit to an exercise program. "In my experience, however, younger people tend to be the least realistic. I get a lot of clients in their 20s and 30s. They think that with enough exercise they can sculpt their bodies and turn into Wonder Woman or Superman. 'Just tell me what I need to do and I'll do it,' they say. I have to talk them out of weight training every day or spending three hours a day at the gym. I tell them they must avoid injury, but I also want them to avoid burnout!

"Last year I had a woman in her late 30s, Stephanie, who wanted to lose 20 pounds for her friend's wedding six weeks away. We've all heard this before! I gave her my lecture on quick weight loss, how it's mostly water, with some muscle and fat. How lifelong exercise with a healthy diet is the way to lose fat. How quick weight loss is almost always followed by quick weight gain. Stephanie listened patiently, but my lecture went in one ear and out the other. She showed me a chart she had drawn up with her weight loss goals listed for each week. She wanted to lose five pounds the first week, and two and one-half pounds per week after that. Stephanie's diet plan was very restrictive and very complicated: fasting every Monday, 600 calories on Tuesday—you know the kind of diet I'm talking about. 'Just tell me what kind of exercise would be best,' she asked. 'What kind of exercise is best for burning fat?'

"She was looking at me expectantly, pen poised above her chart. I could see she had created a box for exercise on each day, from 6:00 to 8:00 pm. She wanted to fill in those blank lines and get started right away. It looked so good on paper! *Here goes,* I thought to myself, getting ready to lose this new client.

"I told Stephanie how much I admired her drive and commitment, but that I couldn't support a program that could harm her health. I referred her to the nutritionist here at the club for sound weight control advice and suggested a balanced exercise program, incorporating the cardiovascular equipment and weights. 'But you won't be able to exercise if you starve yourself, and you are likely to become injured unless you begin slowly and build gradually.'

"Stephanie was disappointed in my response, but in the end she listened. She even lost 10 pounds and has kept it off this whole year. She looks terrific. You know, five years ago I might have jumped right in and helped her fill out that beautiful chart. Now I know that every client I work with builds my reputation. Bad advice to her would reflect poorly on me. Besides, I get tired of seeing people become frustrated on these crazy diets and seeing them think it's all their fault they can't lose weight when it's the diet that's wrong."

Step 4: Review Previous Exercise Experiences

By now you should understand your client's health concerns and have set realistic fitness goals. You are almost ready to draw up an exercise plan, but before you do, review his exercise history. Discussing previous exercise experiences can help him overcome the false hopes syndrome and planning fallacy, and give you important information for your exercise program design. At this point in your first meeting, you may be discretely checking the clock to be sure you don't run out of time. If you continue working with this client, you will pull more information from his stories. However, during the first meeting, your goal is to uncover two things: What works for him, and what doesn't work for him.

What Works?

Ask clients what has worked in the past. What factors have helped them stick to their exercise programs? If they are fairly new to exercise, this discussion may be brief. But some clients have tried many times to start exercise programs, stuck with them for a while, then something happened to interrupt their adherence.

Start by asking about the factors that helped your clients stick to their exercise intentions. What did they like best about previous exercise programs? Encourage them to talk about their positive experiences. How could these be replicated in their new exercise programs? If people can't remember anything positive, ask if they felt good after working out (if the workouts themselves did not feel good). Did they notice that they had more energy during the day? Did they sleep better at night? Did they feel more relaxed? Try to pull out positive experiences even if your clients have difficulty remembering anything positive.

Ask your clients to describe their most successful attempts at regular exercise. Maybe they were most successful when exercising at a particular time of day or at a convenient location. Maybe they walked with a friend, or a four-legged friend. Were they more successful attending a class? Exercising on their own? Did they enjoy sports, but find machines boring? Have they tried listening to music or reading while working out?

Social support may have helped your clients stick to their exercise programs. The word *social* in social support refers not only to family and friends, but also to casual acquaintances and coworkers. Members of an exercise class often serve as social support for one another. Ask clients about ways to improve social support for the exercise program they are about to begin.

As you talk with your clients about positive exercise experiences and what has worked in the past, take careful notes. If you continue to work with a client, you can use these over time to increase her motivation. Although this first discussion will be brief, incorporate useful suggestions into your exercise program design. What worked before may work again. In addition, revisiting positive exercise experiences helps build your client's confidence in her ability to stick to an exercise program. Bolstering your client's self-confidence is extremely important in the early days of an exercise program. The next chapter discusses building self-confidence and self-efficacy.

What Doesn't Work?

As you talk about previous experiences with exercise, clients usually list lots of reasons why previous programs did not work. Some of these may be excuses (I lost my membership card). Others are challenges that were too difficult to overcome (my job moved me to a new building with no fitness facility). Which of these factors could affect the new exercise program? Help clients anticipate possible barriers to exercise and come up with problem-solving strategies. Perhaps you can set up a better exercise program this time around. And by anticipating problems, your clients will be mentally and emotionally prepared to cope.

Some of the things your clients mention at this point in your conversation should prompt you to take a second look at the exercise program you are planning.

- "The exercise program was too difficult." If clients say that their last programs were too difficult or caused a lot of discomfort, get the details of those programs. Some clients have difficulty tolerating exercise that is highly intense or even moderately high in intensity. Instead of trying to teach them to tough it out, prescribe exercise that is moderately intense and or even light in an appropriate volume in the beginning. You want them to walk out of their exercise sessions feeling energized and refreshed, not discouraged and exhausted.

- "I got injured." Ask about the injury. This injury may act up again if the area is weak. For example, an ankle sprained a long time ago may still be weak. Previous overuse injuries, such as shin splints or tendinitis, may be likely to recur. Be sure your exercise program will not overstress these areas, and advise clients to watch for early signs that they should change their exercise routine or cut back.

- "The exercise program took too much time." How much time did it take? What's different about the new program? Either your new program must take less time, or your clients must figure out how to make more time for exercise. Either way, make the program as convenient as you can.

- "Life got too complicated." Many causes of relapse fall under the heading "life got too complicated." Most of your clients have things in their lives besides their exercise programs. Exercise programs are interrupted from time to time by things such as illness, family problems, holidays, travel, bad weather, and too much to do at work or at home. Help clients acknowledge that interruptions are a fact of life. Too often, interruptions lead to attrition. Instead, help clients make a plan for returning to exercise as soon as possible, or for exercising in a different way when time is limited. If you continue working with new clients, work extensively on relapse prevention during the first few months of an exercise program.

Q&A

Q This is a lot of discussion to squeeze into my first session with a new client. How do you fit it all in?

A You may not be able to, so do the most important things first, and do what you have time for without rushing. Your first session should feel comfortable to your clients. They want to feel that you are listening and that you are really interested in them. It is better to cover less material and have a good session than to cover everything in a rush that leaves them feeling confused. Gather preliminary information before your first meeting if possible: medical history, fitness goals, exercise history, and a readiness to exercise questionnaire. Review these before the meeting. Many personal trainers require clients to attend three to five sessions to get started. You can see why. The first session will be mostly talk, covering much of the material in this chapter. Other sessions can include talk during the workout, talk that is both motivational and informational in nature. Whatever you do, never lose sight of the fact that the quality of the time you spend with clients during this first meeting is more important than the quantity of material that you cover.

Step 5: Work With Your Client to Finalize the Exercise Program Design

At this point in your meeting you should have a pretty good idea of what you want to recommend for your client. Use all of the information you have gathered to work with your client to draw up a great exercise program. Clients should be able to see clearly that the program reflects their health concerns, fitness goals, exercise preferences, and all of the other information you have collected. The more input from your client the better as you finalize the exercise program design. Let your client select activities (perhaps from your suggestions) and arrange a workable schedule.

Write the exercise program on a card or calendar that allows clients to record their workouts and track their progress. If more meetings are planned, let them know you will check the cards periodically to see how they are doing.

Remind clients that their first and most important goal is to establish an exercise habit. It is the force of habit that turns an exercise program into a lifetime of regular physical activity. Do everything you can to make the exercise enjoyable and convenient.

Step 6: Help Clients Anticipate the First Day

Before ending the first meeting with a new client, ask him to imagine the next step: getting to his first exercise session. Is he ready to begin? Does he have everything he needs? Does he know where he is going? Does he need more information?

If your client is new to the fitness center where she will work out, give her advice about how to fit in. Information on what to wear, where to change, and even where to stand in a class can be helpful. Beginners often feel awkward in a group with more experienced members.

Many clients benefit from practicing visualization exercises that call on them to use their imaginations for increasing their motivation and problem-solving skills. Your new client is probably too wound up to relax right now, and it usually takes several sessions with a trainer before a client is comfortable enough to enjoy visualization exercises. Nevertheless, you can encourage him to imagine what his first workout day will be like and briefly talk about it with you. What will he do before going to his workout? What will he do to get ready to exercise? What could get in the way? How will he deal with obstacles that might arise?

In your first meeting you have helped your client start thinking about the best ways to stick to an exercise program. In your next meeting you will follow up on many of these ideas, seeds you planted at the first meeting. Send your client off with motivational reading on subjects you think she will be interested in, being sure to include information on the importance of lifelong exercise and tips for staying with it. Then cross your fingers: You've done all you can for today. Give your words and advice time to sink in, and let the exercise program supply a little magic of its own. Hopefully these will help to give your client the energy and determination to make health and wellness a priority.

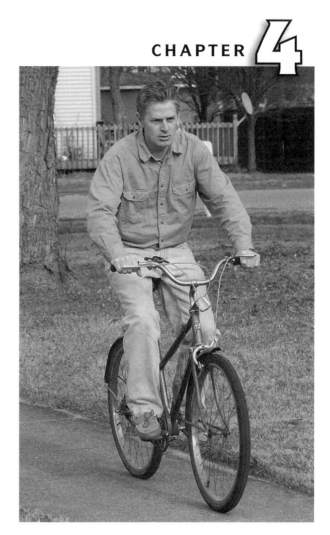

CHAPTER 4

Developing the Force of Habit

You have gotten your clients or patients off to a great start. You have staged them, reviewed health concerns and fitness goals, and helped them devise exercise programs. You have gathered information about their exercise histories that may affect their long-term exercise adherence.

This chapter continues to focus on your early work with clients and patients in the preparation and action stages. As we build on your first meeting, described in the previous chapter, we elaborate on ways to enhance exercise adherence during the first few weeks of an exercise program.

Unless your clients or patients are long-term maintenance exercisers, you can assume that their exercise commitment is fragile at this point. Your job in the preparation and action stages is to continue to educate your clients about exercise benefits and to encourage them to make detailed and realistic exercise plans. Your goal is to strengthen their commitment to their exercise programs and to help them develop behavior change skills that will support their commitment to lifelong exercise.

This chapter discusses the importance of turning exercise into a habit. The force of habit requires fewer decisions and less self-control, which results in fewer opportunities to decide to exercise some other time. This chapter also discusses self-management skills that increase the likelihood of sticking to an exercise program.

Understanding self-efficacy will allow you to help clients believe they can become regular exercisers. *Physical activity self-efficacy* refers to people's perceptions of their ability to perform physical activities and stick to exercise programs. Physical activity self-efficacy is a strong predictor of exercise success; therefore, this chapter suggests ways to enhance your clients' exercise self-efficacy. Strong self-efficacy helps clients continue to strive for regular physical activity even in the face of difficulties that might otherwise cause them to throw in the towel. This chapter also briefly reviews the importance of social support systems and how to encourage clients to develop the social support that will help them stick to an exercise program.

The chapter ends with a review of behavior change skills essential for continued exercise adherence. Psychologists call these *self-management skills* because they help people manage their thoughts, feelings, and behavior in ways that support behavior change goals.

Force of Habit and the Nature of Self-Control

We are creatures of habit. Our habits carry us through the day, providing a comfortable routine that gives us a base for facing challenges. Psychologists believe that we can tolerate only a relatively small amount of disruption to our routines before experiencing stress (Vohs and Heatherton 2000).

When clients and patients begin exercise programs, they must change their routines to accommodate this new activity. Changing our routines requires the ability to cope with the resulting stress. Because coping requires energy, it takes energy to change a habit, such as beginning an exercise program or changing eating habits. Your clients might refer to this energy as *willpower.* Psychologists call it *self-regulation* or *self-control* (Muraven, Tice, and Baumeister 1998).

Self-control refers to the control people exert over their thoughts, emotions, and behaviors. When making decisions and choices, initiating and inhibiting behavior, and making and carrying out plans, we draw on self-control. We use self-control when we forgo immediate pleasure (lying on the couch and reading) in order to obtain future benefits (better health). Self-control allows us to examine and change habitual behavior.

If you have worked with people for a while, you have observed that self-control varies widely from person to person. Some have a great deal of resolve and determination, and others seem to be thrown off by the slightest challenge.

Psychologists who have studied self-control believe it is a limited resource (Baumeister et al. 1998; Giner-Sorolla 2001; Muraven and Baumeister 2000; Vohs and Heatherton 2000). Each person has a limited amount of psychic energy to expend on self-control. Some have more, and some have less, but each person has a limited amount. This notion of limitation helps explain why people who exercise early in the morning have the highest success rates; they have not yet expended time and energy overcoming the barriers that inevitably develop during the day. This concept of limitation may also explain why dieters are most likely to overeat in the evening. After exerting self-control all day to resist temptation, their resolve wears down by the end of the day.

The good news is that practicing self-control appears to strengthen self-control ability (Muraven and Baumeister 2000). As we practice delaying gratification for future well-being, we get better at doing so. That's why parents and educational systems spend time helping kids develop self-control in the form of self-discipline. The more you practice, the better you get.

The bad news is that coping with stress reduces the energy available for self-control. This helps explain why stress often causes people to quit exercising, to resume smoking and other addictive behaviors, or to go off their diets. When stress uses up our limited supply of self-control energy, resolve goes down the drain (Baumeister et al. 1998). But more good news: Exercise improves people's ability to cope with stress. So once clients make the exercise–stress reduction connection, they may find that exercise reduces stress and helps them stick to their exercise programs.

Q&A

Q Do you think that habitual exercisers (people in the maintenance stage of exercise behavior) have more self-control than others?

A It is true that many regular exercisers also have pretty good self-control when it comes to other health habits, such as diet. But just because they exhibit self-control when it comes to exercise, this doesn't necessarily mean they have more self-control in all areas. On the other hand, you may meet clients in the preparation and action stages who have excellent self-control in some areas of their lives, such as work or parenting, but have little energy to spare for exercise. The challenge is to help them set up programs of physical activity that require minimal self-control because they may be energy depleted. In light of the research on self-control it is easy to see why those in maintenance actually attend and complete their workouts. For one thing, just as you suggest, these people may have had greater amounts of self-control to begin with. For another, exercise has become a habit that requires less self-control than it did when they first began to exercise. And, these clients may have developed additional self-control during their years of exercising. Finally, most people in maintenance are firm believers in the stress reducing power of exercise. Stress may throw them for a day or two, but as believers, they are likely to eventually return to their exercise programs in order to restore their emotional equilibrium.

We've said before that fitness professionals are sometimes guilty of designing fitness programs that look great on paper, but don't match the amount of energy clients are able or willing to expend. This is partly because clients themselves don't really understand what they can realistically take on and underestimate the time and energy an exercise program will require. To improve your new clients' fitness success rates, try to help them maximize their motivation and self-control energy, while reducing the amount of self-control their exercise programs will require, by using the following suggestions.

Remind Clients That Exercise Programs Require Time and Energy

Sometimes we are tempted to downplay the time and energy that regular physical activity requires. We may be afraid we will scare clients away if exercise programs sound too demanding or difficult. But it is important to remind clients that even though regular exercise delivers enormous rewards, it also requires time and energy. Ask clients to tell you what they are realistically willing to do. Ask them to make a commitment. They will realize they must strengthen their resolve and be prepared for the challenges that lie ahead. People who mentally prepare for the demands of taking on a program of regular physical activity are better able to summon the self-control required to be successful.

Encourage Clients to Make Their Health a Priority

Unless clients believe that their long-term health is a priority, other commitments will consume the time and energy they could be spending on physical activity. During your first meetings, you reviewed your clients' health concerns. Remind clients that regular exercise is essential for preventing or treating the concerns they mentioned. Remind them also that they should never take their health for granted and that good health is a prerequisite for achieving other important goals: performing work, caring for family, and participating in other high-priority activities. When exercise is a priority, people will exert more self-control to make room for it in their lives.

Design an Exercise Program That Can Quickly Become a Habit

Once exercise becomes a habitual routine, little self-control is required. Use this force of habit to increase fitness success. Clients can usually tell you how they can fit exercise into their days. Always let clients take the lead when setting up exercise times and locations. Make the exercise program as convenient as possible. A "same time, same place" kind of routine is the best way to establish an exercise habit, although there are many variations on this theme. Shoot for simplicity, especially for clients new to exercise and for clients still in preparation or action/ambivalent stages. Keep the exercise program easy to follow and short. Once clients establish a simple exercise habit, you can increase the exercise volume. You are kind of like a drug dealer here: You want to be sure you get your client hooked!

Suggest Early-Morning Exercise

Research shows that people who exercise first thing in the morning are generally the most successful in sticking to their exercise programs. It is easier to exert self-control early in the day before other demands require your energy. Therefore, when your clients work out first thing in the morning, they will accomplish their goals before other demands eat up their time and wear away their self-control energy supply.

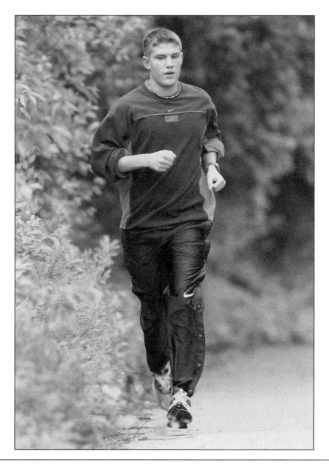

Early-morning exercise and outdoor exercise can help your clients develop a routine and reduce stress.

Encourage Clients to Find Stress-Reducing Benefits in Their Exercise Programs

Just as people learn to overeat to reduce stress, so can they learn to exercise to reduce stress, a much more helpful response! Educate clients about the stress reducing benefits of regular exercise, and encourage them to exercise when they feel tense. When clients learn to use exercise to reduce stress, three benefits result: They reduce feelings of stress, they create an additional incentive to exercise regularly, and they increase their self-control energy. It's a win-win-win situation!

Suggest That Clients Invite Friends to Join Them

Social support reduces the need for self-control. Working out with a friend makes it more difficult to decide not to exercise because you don't want to disappoint your friend who is waiting for you. Instead of wasting energy thinking up excuses, you put on your sneakers and head for the gym.

Thinking up excuses depletes self-control energy. Imagine that you feel like skipping your workout today. If you are going to your workout alone, you start weighing the pros and cons, thinking about all the other things you have to do, and about how tired you are. You start feeling stressed about the demands in your life right now, and pretty soon you feel exhausted and overwhelmed and decide to skip the workout.

But what if a friend is waiting for you? You don't have time for the negative thoughts and deliberations. You are out the door in a flash, and you start feeling better once you see your friend and start to exercise. You didn't waste energy on self-control, and the exercise reduced your stress level.

Build Self-Efficacy

Self-efficacy refers to a person's belief in his or her ability to perform a given task. Self-efficacy is a central concept in social cognitive theory, formulated by Albert Bandura (1982, 1987). Social cognitive theory predicts that people are more likely to engage in a given behavior, such as regular exercise, if they think they can and if they expect it to deliver positive benefits.

Self-efficacy is similar to self-confidence, except that self-efficacy is always situation- or behavior-specific. For example, you might have high self-efficacy in your ability to walk regularly, but low-self efficacy in your ability to stick to a strength training program.

Many studies have found that exercise self-efficacy is a good predictor of whether or not people will stick to their exercise programs. Strong self-efficacy helps clients strive for regular physical activity in the face of obstacles. Perhaps you have observed this in your own work. If early in your working relationship with clients they voice uncertainty about their abilities to stick to exercise programs, you are probably right in foreseeing early dropout or difficulties.

Can you do anything to strengthen a client's self-efficacy? And do these interventions work? Several studies have explored these questions, and the answer to both is yes (McAuley and Blissmer 2000). The following techniques for improving self-efficacy hold the most promise and seem to have the greatest potential to increase exercise adherence (Schlicht, Godin, and Camaione 1999).

Help Clients Be Immediately Successful

The best way to increase feelings of self-efficacy is to show clients that they can do it, whatever "it" is. Accomplishing a task or acquiring a new skill is called *performance mastery* (Schlicht, Godin, and Camaione 1999) or *mastery accomplishments* (McAuley et al. 1994). As clients master the skills required to stick to exercise programs, their self-efficacy grows. They see themselves performing the skills, realize what they have accomplished, then start believing they can continue.

Take a look at your clients. What activity could they successfully accomplish early to demonstrate that they are successful? False praise won't cut it. Clients must set small goals for themselves and believe that they have achieved them. The goal could be learning to use a piece of equipment, coming to the fitness center twice a week, learning how to fill in the workout card, or whatever would be the most obvious next step in acquiring an exercise habit.

Self-efficacy is all about perception; your clients must *perceive* themselves as successful. You may have to spell this out for them when setting fitness goals. Break large goals into smaller, easily achievable goals. Make lists that your clients see and check off goals as they are achieved. Adjust these goals as you get to know your clients or patients better, making them easier or more difficult as necessary.

The key to setting your clients up for success is to accurately judge their abilities, so that you can ask them to achieve the achievable. Even then, although they are successful in your eyes, they may not see it that way. To increase their feelings of self-efficacy you may have to help them overcome deep-seated misconceptions about what it means to be successful. You may have to discuss their (possibly unrealistic) expectations and ideas about exercise behavior and fitness goals. Use performance mastery in conjunction with the other techniques described in this section.

Expose Clients to Role Models Similar to Themselves

When clients see someone similar to themselves performing the task in question, they think, *If that person can do it, so can I!* The key is finding people similar enough to your clients or patients that they identify with them. To do this, you must uncover the defining variables that, in their eyes, limit their ability to be successful. This could be age, gender, ethnicity, sedentary background, class, ability level, body type, and so forth. Your clients will usually provide clues: "I don't want to be the oldest one in the class," or "I'm afraid I'll be the only out-of-shape person in the fitness center."

Where do you find role models? Wherever you can! Real people are best if you can find other clients, fitness professionals, friends, or acquaintances who can be seen working out or doing whatever it is you want your clients to do. If you are lucky you might be able to find a group that caters to your client's limitation, for example, a class for older adults or people new to exercise. If you think there is a market, you could start a program for this group and recruit others. This is doubly powerful because you wrap up social support and role modeling in one neat package. If the group leader could belong to this group, you get triple power.

If you can't find real people to serve as role models, loan out videotapes designed for that group, or books and articles showing people similar to your client engaged in regular exercise. Tell her about similar clients you have worked with who have been successful in their exercise programs. Share newspapers and magazine stories about similar people. For example, *Arthritis Today,* published by the Arthritis Foundation, includes stories in most issues about people with arthritis who manage to exercise regularly. You can find more information on www.arthritis.org.

Help Clients Recruit an Exercise Partner

Social support enhances self-efficacy, just as it enhances exercise adherence, in many ways. Your client might have a family member, friend, or acquaintance who would like to join him. Provide him an incentive, financial or otherwise, to join your program with a friend. Many personal trainers can work with two people at a time, as long as exercise goals, fitness levels, and exercise programs are similar. Most of the time, exercise partners tell each other how well they are doing and remind each other to come to their next workout. People see themselves reflected by their partners. "My exercise partner seems to think I am doing it. I must be doing it."

Provide Education
and Positive Reinforcement

People with low exercise self-efficacy greatly doubt their exercise abilities. Therefore, they often need more reassurance than others that they are performing exercises correctly. Give them the information they need so that they feel they are doing it right. Be patient as you reassure them they are feeling the exercise in the right place, or that it is normal to feel somewhat out of breath at the correct exercise intensity.

Positive reinforcement strengthens clients' exercise self-efficacy. Positive reinforcement is best provided with mastery experiences. Rewards, such as free personal training sessions, are also reinforcing. Concrete signs of progress toward goals are strong reinforcements. Help clients see improvements wherever they can.

Your spoken reinforcement is also helpful. Most helpful is concrete, positive feedback, pointing out exactly what your clients have done well, or improvements you have noticed. Instead of telling them that they are looking better or doing better, you might say that they look more energetic or that they are accomplishing more in their workouts.

Help Clients Look Good

Self-efficacy judgments are often (and erroneously) based on appearance. If possible, and as tactfully as possible, help clients new to exercise find apparel that allows them to move and is flattering. Without sounding critical or overstepping the bounds of etiquette, mention what people usually wear where they will exercise. This will help them feel like they fit in when they show up their first day. Nothing lowers self-efficacy for new exercisers than feeling embarrassed about the way they look.

Social Physique Anxiety

Many of your clients low in exercise self-efficacy may experience anxiety about appearing in public in exercise clothing. Social physique anxiety occurs when a client worries that others are appraising his body. This anxiety may make a client reluctant to join an exercise class or work out in a fitness center, or even go for a walk in public. Social physique anxiety may go along with a distorted body image, so that even very good-looking people may still feel too fat and worry about how they look.

It's easy to see where this anxiety comes from. After all, people do check each other out in fitness settings, or any place for that matter. We judge other people based on how they look. We think to ourselves, "That person in the grocery line shouldn't be buying that cake," and "That guy is too old to be running."

How can you best work with clients who experience social physique anxiety? You can try to reassure them that many people's bodies are far from perfect and that what other people think is unimportant. Give advice on finding comfortable and flattering exercise apparel. If your center has a shop that sells apparel, stock flattering styles. If clients are willing to go to a fitness center, they may prefer slow times with fewer patrons. If they refuse to exercise in public, they may wish to use exercise equipment or videotapes at home. If body image appears to be a big issue that is significantly interfering with a client's life, recommend professional help.

Social Support: Helping Relationships

We humans are social animals, and the activities and opinions of our social network strongly influence our behavior and beliefs. People with strong social support fare better in many areas, and behavior change programs are no exception. Friends, family, coworkers, and other people provide company, encouragement, resources, and support. In fact, social support is one of the strongest predictors of exercise adherence and fitness success.

Research on behavior change suggests that social support increases exercise adherence in many ways. First of all, social support provides emotional support, such as encouragement and praise. Social support helps clients feel they are doing the right thing. As stated earlier, social support increases exercise self-efficacy. Second, social support can include an exercise partner, who "forces" clients to show up even when clients don't feel like exercising. Third, social support provides logistical support, enabling the client to participate in an exercise program. For example, a client may be able to use her lunch hour for exercise because her work environment is supportive. One spouse may be able to work out early in the morning because the other gets the children off to school.

We learned earlier in this chapter that social support, in the form of an exercise partner, can reduce the need for self-control and spare self-control energy. In addition, we often use social support to reduce stress, which in turn helps us stick to exercise programs. Simply talking to others and voicing our concerns reduces feelings of stress. And talking our problems over with others gives us a chance to find new ways to deal with the sources of stress.

You may already have discussed social support in your first meeting with a new client if you talked about what contributed to his previous fitness success. People often mention that at one time they were regular exercisers because they had workout buddies or walked regularly with family members or friends.

If social support does not come up in your first meeting, bring it up soon thereafter. You might ask a question such as, "Can you think of ways your family and friends can help you stick to your exercise program?" Listen carefully to ideas that come up.

For some clients, social support may already be quite strong. Others may have a limited number of connections. Do your clients take advantage of possible support sources? Would they like to ask family members or friends to exercise with them? If they exercise during the workday, would colleagues like to join them? If they have trouble sticking to an exercise program, could family or friends help? Brainstorm and explore the possibilities.

Some of your clients may have little social support. They may have no family, a disinterested family, or few friends interested in physical activity. If it sounds like there are no friends or colleagues waiting in the wings for an exercise opportunity, you may need to help your clients find support at the fitness center or through their work with you. Don't forget, you can be a strong and effective source of social support. You may also be able to create opportunities at your fitness center that encourage interaction and social support among members (Annesi 2002b). For example, some fitness centers set up mentoring programs that partner experienced exercisers with new members to help new members feel at home. Or you might form informal groups of new members for orientation programs, welcome receptions, or whatever seems to make sense for your center and its programs. Special small classes for new exercisers can provide comfort and a nonthreatening environment for those who feel awkward and out of place in the fitness center. If you are a group exercise instructor, take time to introduce new students to each other.

Q&A

Q You say social support is extremely important for exercise adherence, but I have had several clients who really enjoyed exercising alone.

A Many people do enjoy exercising alone. In fact, they may use their exercise time to get away from people, or at least to be alone in a crowd. They don't want to talk to anyone or be slowed by other people. They may not want to meet new people at the fitness center or serve as mentors. That is fine. Respect their need for solitude and privacy, and do not force group participation upon them. Remember that social support comes in many forms. People who like to exercise alone may have terrific social support at work or at home that enables them to exercise regularly. Colleagues at work may cover the phone while your client is working out. Family members may be home cooking dinner or watching the kids.

Animal lovers know that no discussion of social support would be complete without a brief mention of our beloved pets. While we have known a few cats who will go for a walk, we must admit that the dogs really win the exercise program support contest. Dogs encourage a great deal of physical activity; they need daily walks to stay healthy and can cajole their owners into active play. Many people walk long distances each day with their dogs and enjoy taking them hiking. Dogs are happy, supportive companions who reduce their owners' stress with their unconditional adoration, while helping them stay healthy with regular exercise. What a great combination! Encourage clients who love their dogs to make the most of this wonderful exercise opportunity.

Behavior Change Skills

Behavior change skills include a variety of self-management techniques that clients use to support their behavior change efforts. *Self-management* refers to managing your behavior, thoughts, and emotions. Self-management skills improve your ability to look at your behavior, thoughts, and emotions objectively and to change things that need changing. They help you cope effectively with stress and adapt to lifestyle changes, such as those that occur when beginning an exercise program. Behavior change skills help you develop a habit and strengthen self-control.

How do you manage behavior, thoughts, and emotions? You manage your behavior when you set up an exercise program that is easy to follow and when you schedule exercise into your day. You manage your thoughts and feelings by the way you see life and by the way you talk to yourself. When you feel stressed, you take action to deal with the source of stress and you do something (get some exercise!) to calm yourself.

Effective self-management skills maximize self-control energy, channeling it into the most important areas. Self-management skills increase the likelihood that desired changes in behavior will occur. These skills help clients change their environments in ways that support their exercise program adherence and help clients cope with difficulties that might otherwise short-circuit plans to exercise regularly.

Where do effective self-management skills come from? Unfortunately, they are rarely taught, unless a client has had experience with stress management training or helpful counseling. Some clients practice many of these self-management skills intuitively. For example, some clients seem to have a natural ability to maintain a positive attitude and to talk themselves into exercising even when they don't feel like it. Fortunately, many self-management skills are actually common sense, and their applications to exercise adherence are easily taught. You probably practice many of them yourself, although you may never have called them self-management skills.

Effective self-management skills enhance the likelihood of success in any behavior change program. The following skills have been found most helpful for improving exercise adherence.

Self-Monitoring

Self-monitoring usually takes the form of a daily written record of the behavior you are trying to change. People trying to establish an exercise habit can keep exercise logs. Most clients prefer a log that is fairly small, portable, and easy to understand. Be sure there is enough room for a complete record of each workout. Clients may want to use a workout card for their strength training sessions. They may wish to record time, calories expended, exercise heart rate, or other variables for cardio-vascular exercise. Some clients may simply wish to record the activity and the number of minutes spent in that activity. In general, detailed information is beneficial if it indicates progress over time, for example, an increase in the resistance on strength training equipment. But the act of recording seems to be more important than the method used for recording, so if your clients prefer something simple, that is fine (Baker and Kirschenbaum 1998).

Self-monitoring increases exercise adherence for several reasons. For one thing, if clients use exercise logs to demonstrate what they have done between personal training sessions with you, they will be motivated to exercise so that they will have impressive records to show you. The exercise log becomes more important if someone else looks at it.

Logging a workout serves as a reward, encouraging clients or patients to stick to their programs. Regular adherence is the most important component of fitness success in the first few weeks of an exercise program, and these logs represent their achievements. Clients are proud of the accomplishments recorded in their logs. I once had a client who kept a monthly calendar on her desk dedicated to recording workouts. She recorded her workouts in pen, and then with highlighters color coded the different types of exercise. She highlighted twice-weekly strength workouts in yellow. She highlighted her bicycle rides in green (she was training for a long-distance ride a few months away), and other cardiovascular activity in purple. The colorful mosaic that slowly emerged over the month became a delightful testimony to her fitness success.

Self-monitoring encourages clients to stick to their exercise programs because it encourages honest self-evaluation. It's easy to make vague, self-reassuring statements like, "I exercise fairly regularly," or "It won't hurt if I skip my exercise session today," or "I think I've been to the fitness center several times this month." But when the workout calendar has two weeks of blank days it's more difficult to feel reassured. It's like a mirror, reflecting an image of your exercise activity. Your workout record tells you in no-nonsense black-and-white terms where you stand on your exercise program attendance.

Self-monitoring also helps you find solutions to problems by helping you and your clients identify situations and events that interfere with their exercise programs. Let's say you have been working with a client for several weeks, and his exercise logs show that his plans to walk on the weekend rarely come to fruition. Is weekend exercise not realistic for him? What if he walked first thing in the morning instead of trying to squeeze it in before dinner, as originally planned? Or would he rather do something besides walk?

Provide your clients exercise logs at the first session. As time goes by, elicit their feedback about what works and what doesn't work with their logs, and encourage them to find effective self-monitoring systems.

Q&A

Q How important is accuracy for clients keeping exercise logs? And what do you do about sloppy logs?

A According to research, when it comes to adherence, record-keeping accuracy is not extremely important. The act of keeping a log is more important than keeping an accurate log. If a client records that she stretched for 10 minutes and she only stretched for 8, do not fret. However, if certain variables recorded in the log are used to measure progress, then accuracy becomes more important. For example, if you tell your clients to look for changes in resting heart rate, then the conditions under which resting heart rate is taken are extremely important. Encourage clients to strive for accuracy if the measurements are important. As for sloppy logs, personal trainers get pretty good at reading all kinds of handwriting. And as long as your clients can read their own writing and are happy with their record keeping, then sloppiness does not get in the way.

Stimulus Control

Stimulus control is psychology jargon for controlling the factors that affect the behavior you want to change. Naturally, you want to control these factors in ways that promote desirable change. Stimulus control has also been called *contingency control.*

Stimulus control is based on the observation that certain factors stimulate predictable responses in each of us. For some people, going into a bar for a beer means it's time to light up a cigarette. Watching a movie might be a signal to eat candy or popcorn. Once people identify a stimulus that causes a problematic behavior, they can begin to change or eliminate the stimulus, or at least plan a new response (Prochaska, Johnson, and Lee 1998).

What factors stimulate sedentary behavior and cause people to shelve their plans to exercise? Something as simple as not being able to find their workout clothes can interfere with some people's exercise plans. A special television show may tempt clients to stay glued to the tube. Rainy weather can cancel outdoor exercise, or a sick child home from school might mean no trip to the fitness center for the caretaker. Friends coming over for dinner may cause some to rush home early, skipping their late afternoon workouts.

Clients are usually pretty good at identifying what kinds of situations and events keep them from exercising as planned. Their exercise logs may also provide clues. Help your clients think of ways to cope with these events and situations, especially the ones that occur frequently.

Success Story

Success Story: Simple Solutions

Nate, a personal trainer, had a client, Will, who was disorganized. Disorganized people can find it difficult to set up an exercise habit, and Will was no exception. As Nate worked with Will to figure out why he often skipped his exercise sessions, he uncovered several simple problems that were easily solved. One of these was having exercise clothes readily available in several locations. Sometimes Will needed his workout clothes at home, and other times he needed them in the car so he could work out at the fitness center on the way home from work. The solution? Will bought another set of clothes, including shoes, and kept them in the car so that he didn't need to remember workout clothes on the days he would exercise on his way home. Will's adherence improved significantly when his need for flexibility was met.

You can help clients develop cues that remind them to exercise. The exercise log itself is a reminder to stick to an exercise program. Other cues might be written reminders posted at key locations at home and at work. Exercise clothes laid out the night before help people get to morning exercise classes. A past photo from fitter and thinner days posted on the refrigerator can reinforce the resolve to stick to an exercise program.

Reinforcement Management and Counterconditioning

The idea behind reinforcement management is this: Behaviors that are rewarded are more likely to be performed again. Therefore, be sure you do not reward counterproductive behavior (skipping an exercise session), and be sure to reward productive behavior (sticking to the exercise program). The key is to help clients find an immediate reward for their exercise participation. Do whatever you can to help them craft an exercise program that is as enjoyable and rewarding as it can be.

Your clients or patients having trouble sticking to an exercise program may find a technique called *counterconditioning* helpful. Counterconditioning is trying to change a conditioned response to a particular situation and it focuses more on unproductive habits than on occasional problems.

For example, if you always smoke while you make phone calls, try to replace smoking with drawing on scrap paper to keep your hands busy. Help your clients figure out new responses to the situations that keep them from exercising.

Success Story
An Alternative Approach

How might counterconditioning apply in an exercise situation? Here's an example. Erin had a personal training client, Kim, who liked to walk with her friend, Angela, who lived down the street. But Angela was often busy and would call to say she couldn't walk as planned. Kim's conditioned (habitual) response? She wouldn't walk either. Erin wanted to help her come up with a new response to this situation. She suggested that Kim go ahead and walk by herself, but Kim felt unsafe walking alone. Erin suggested that she work out using an exercise video during the time she would have been walking with her friend. Erin helped her choose a video with music and a style of exercise she enjoyed, and Kim began to substitute the video exercise for simply giving up on exercise altogether. She still enjoyed walking with Angela, but on the days that Angela canceled, Kim popped in the video and exercised at home.

The goals of stimulus control, reinforcement management, and counterconditioning are all the same. They are simply fancy terms for slightly different approaches to getting rid of bad habits and forming new ones. Remember, the sooner exercise becomes a habit, the less self-control is required and the easier it is for your clients to stick to their exercise programs.

The Transtheoretical Model and the Processes of Change

A great deal of psychological research has looked at how people change their behaviors. The stages of change model presented in chapter 2 is part of a larger theory known as the transtheoretical model (TTM) of behavior change (Prochaska, Johnson, and Lee 1998). TTM is one of the most widely used models to have grown out of this body of research. One idea from TTM is that people use various processes to help themselves change their behaviors and progress through the stages of change. These processes have been referred to as the *processes of change* (Prochaska and Velicer

(continued)

(continued)

1997).This chapter discusses the processes most related to changing exercise behavior, drawn from a variety of behavior change models.Table 4.1 describes the processes of change from the transtheoretical model. More information on applying these processes of change to physical activity can be found in the works of Courneya and Bobick (2000), Marcus and Simkin (1994), and Prochaska, Johnson, and Lee (1998).

The processes of change are divided into two groups (table 4.1).The processes classified as cognitive/experiential refer to the ways in which people's behavior changes as a result of changing the way they think and changing the way they view their lives and the world around them.The processes classified as behavioral/environmental refer to the ways that people modify their environments and change their behavior in response to these changes in the environment. In psychology, environment refers to people as well as physical surroundings. Researchers have found that the cognitive/experiential processes are more common in helping people move through the early stages of behavior change (some of these were discussed in chapter 3), while the behavioral processes are more commonly used by people moving from preparation to action, and from action to maintenance (Prochaska and Marcus 1994).

Table 4.1
Processes of Change

Cognitive/Experiential	
1. Consciousness-raising	Seeking more information and increasing one's awareness about exercise and exercise benefits
2. Emotional relief	Feeling good about deciding to change sedentary behavior, thereby relieving distress regarding sedentary behavior
3. Self-reevaluation	Evaluating one's self-image based on the value of physical activity and the importance of including exercise in one's life
4. Social reevaluation	Accepting a change in self-concept regarding one's social role, e.g., a change in self-concept from a sedentary individual to an active individual, and everything this change in role implies
5. Self-liberation	Choosing to change, and believing that one can change, despite one's roles as perceived by others

Behavioral/Environmental	
6. Stimulus control	Controlling situations and cues that trigger sedentary behavior
7. Counterconditioning	Substitution of physical activity for sedentary responses to certain cues
8. Reinforcement management	Changing the factors that reinforce sedentary behavior; adding reinforcements for exercise behavior
9. Helping relationships	Developing social support from family, friends, and acquaintances for one's participation in physical activity
10. Environmental reevaluation	Thinking about the impact one's sedentary behavior has on one's family, friends, and other people

Managing Stress and Negative Emotions

The previous section stated that stress is the most common reason people quit their exercise programs. Stress depletes energy that could otherwise be used for self-control, leaving us emotionally exhausted and without the energy to get to workouts or resist the temptation to smoke or overeat.

In addition to using up energy, stress can also trigger negative emotions, such as anger and sadness. When people experience negative feelings, or distress, they look for ways to feel better. The need to overcome distress is perceived as more important than behaving in ways that may result in future benefits (Tice, Bratslavsky, and Baumeister 2001). If you feel bad and think skipping your workout will make you feel better, you will skip the workout, even though you would like to get back in shape.

You can help your clients stick to their exercise programs by talking about the importance of managing stress and negative emotions. Help them figure out simple ways to cope with negative emotions and to reduce feelings of stress that can accumulate throughout the day and cause them to neglect their exercise programs. Most clients already understand what causes stress in their lives and the different ways they cope with it. Of course, some ways of coping are more productive than others; help clients think about which coping skills work best for them. Suggest simple ways to reduce stress and negative emotions, so that these feelings will not disrupt your clients' exercise programs.

Stress management techniques fall into two categories (Lazarus and Folkman 1984). The first is problem-focused coping. You use problem-focused coping when you identify the problem, then look for solutions. The second is emotion-focused coping. You use emotion-focused coping when you engage in activities that help reduce feelings of stress and negative emotions and help you feel better.

Problem Solving: Problem-Focused Coping

The first thing most people do when feeling stressed is try to figure out what causes the stress, and then do something about it (Matheny et al. 1986). Sometimes we come up with ways to eliminate the sources of stress or to at least change them so that they cause less stress. Most clients will not want helpful advice from you about changing their jobs or their marriages, or about dealing with troubled kids, so refrain from trying to solve clients' problems yourself. But if clients complain about stress, you may ask, "What have you tried to do so far?" Encourage an active approach, but let clients solve their own problems or advise them to see a professional if the problems are chronic or causing a lot of disruption.

If the exercise program is a source of stress, then by all means step in and suggest modifications to reduce stress. In this case it is appropriate for you to help clients in the problem solving process.

Emotion-Focused Coping

After people have done as much as they can to address the source of stress (and sometimes there is not much a person can do), they may still feel the need to "change the channel," and take action to reduce feelings of stress. Emotion-focused coping refers to things people do to reduce feelings of stress and improve mood.

Most clients have a pretty good repertoire of stress reduction techniques. Many will mention activities such as talking to friends, taking a walk, listening to music, spending time with their pets, or enjoying hobbies. We often change the channel on stress by doing something we enjoy.

When you mention stress management to clients, they may think of meditation and other exercises that require a great deal of time (which they may not have) and mental discipline. They will be happy to hear that they already practice stress management every day! One of the best ways to reduce feelings of stress is to engage in activities that make us feel good.

Exercise

Exercise is one of the best stress management techniques in the world. It increases feelings of energy and improves mood. It helps relieve feelings of anxiety and depression. The side effects, improved health and appearance, can't be beat. Always ask about stress during your discussions of health concerns and fitness goals, and if stress is a problem, suggest that exercise is the solution.

Healthy Pleasures

Encourage clients to use healthy pleasures to reduce feelings of stress. This type of stress management is easy to teach, and easy to do (Brehm 1998). No special instructions are required. And clients like to hear that they are already experts in stress management (they are!) and that they already practice many helpful techniques to manage stress levels.

I give clients a piece of paper and ask them to list 20 things they enjoy doing. These can be big or little, but at least 10 should be available to the client several times a week. Most clients come up with pretty good lists. Encourage them to think small. Maybe they enjoy a morning cup of tea, a good book before bed, watching the birds, taking their dog for a walk, or watching a funny movie. I then ask clients to select items they would like to use more often for relaxation and enjoyment and to think of ways to use these during the week. See page 84 for a sample worksheet.

Success Story
Healthy Pleasures for Stress Management

Richard has been a water exercise instructor and personal trainer at a community fitness center for eight years. He shared the following story. "Many of my clients are really busy and stressed out. Of course I tell them how exercise will help them feel better and less stressed, and most of them say this is true for them. But some need additional stress reduction techniques. We have stress reduction classes at our center, but of course the really stressed-out clients don't have time to attend. I use the healthy pleasures worksheet with my personal training clients and I also hand it out to the people in my classes. They love the idea of simply becoming more mindful of daily pleasures—it doesn't take any more time. They don't have to attend a class or go on some kind of retreat. It's such a logical idea: You can't feel bad if you feel good! And feeling good is simple and good for you! You can reduce stress by watching the birds, walking your dog, or reading a story to your kid! People put amazing things on their lists I never thought of: watering your plants, looking at photographs of people you love, and remembering happy times.

"I redo the healthy pleasures worksheet myself every so often. You know, our work culture can be so stressful. Everybody is way too serious, and it seems like people think we have to be stressed to be productive and get stuff done. Thank goodness my work allows me to have fun. But even the fitness center environment can be a stressed-out place. It's nuts. We need to remember we are about promoting health, and you can't be healthy if you're stressed out. We fitness instructors have to set an example."

Healthy Pleasures Worksheet

Engaging in healthy pleasures is a great way to reduce feelings of stress. List 20 things you enjoy doing. They can be big or little. At least 10 of these items should be available to you several times a week, preferably every day.

1. _____ 11. _____

2. _____ 12. _____

3. _____ 13. _____

4. _____ 14. _____

5. _____ 15. _____

6. _____ 16. _____

7. _____ 17. _____

8. _____ 18. _____

9. _____ 19. _____

10. _____ 20. _____

Next to each item write how often you use that activity for relaxation and enjoyment.

Circle those you would like to use more often for relaxation and enjoyment.

Write down two changes you could make to take greater advantage of healthy pleasures in your daily life.

Goal 1: _____

_____

Goal 2: _____

_____

Mindful Awareness for Stress Reduction and Relaxation

Some clients may express an interest in more information about stress reduction techniques. Mindful awareness exercises are easy to teach, easy to learn, and very effective in promoting relaxation. *Mindfulness* simply means being totally aware and in the present moment. Your awareness includes not only sensory information but your thoughts and emotions, as well. You are aware as an observer of your thoughts and experiences, which can encourage a deeper understanding of yourself and your problems. While mindfulness is used as a type of meditation, it can also be used in daily activities, such as breathing, eating, and walking. Mindfulness helps you live more fully in the present, and appreciate life with all your senses (Kabat-Zinn 1984).

Mindful awareness, like any relaxation or visualization exercise, is performed most successfully when you try not to try. Once you start trying to achieve mindful awareness, you hamper your ability to relax. Let it go, stop trying, and observe whatever happens.

Mindful Awareness

1. Sit or lie in a comfortable position. Relax for a few minutes, perhaps listening to soothing music.

2. Close your eyes and focus your awareness on the sensory information reaching you at this moment. What sounds do you hear? Are they loud? Soft? Harsh? Smooth? What smells are you aware of? Move your hands over nearby surfaces. What do you feel? As thoughts come and go, simply observe them without becoming involved, and gently turn your attention back to the present moment.

3. Tune in to the sensations within your body: your breathing, your heartbeat, muscle tension, pressure, or any other feelings.

4. Tune back in to sensory input: sounds, smells, tactile sensations.

5. Open your eyes and notice what you see. Pretend you are seeing your surroundings for the first time. Notice shapes, colors, shadows, and composition.

Tuning in to your breathing with mindful awareness can be done throughout the day. For example, you can use the time in your car waiting at a stoplight to bring yourself into the present moment and take a few easy, deep, relaxing breaths. You can breathe mindfully while you wait for your computer to boot up, the toast to pop up, or the water to boil. Waiting in line at the bank or grocery store, or sitting in traffic provide opportunities for mindful awareness, deep breathing, and relaxation.

Q&A

Q I don't have any training in stress management or meditation. Can I still teach relaxation techniques such as mindful awareness or breathing exercises to my clients?

A You will probably be more comfortable giving instruction in these techniques if you take a stress management class or workshop. You may also enjoy reading books about stress management (e.g., Brehm 1998). While these techniques are simple, you need a certain level of confidence to teach them. Observe how other people teach these skills, so that you will see how to present them effectively. You will also be a better teacher if you practice the techniques yourself. Simple techniques such as mindful awareness and deep breathing are safe. If you are a personal trainer or fitness instructor, you can find or make handouts describing these techniques (such as the mindful awareness exercise outlined earlier) and give them to your clients to try, with a brief introduction from you. You may wish to talk clients through these exercises the first time. Clients may have trouble relaxing in a personal training situation, however. Group situations are generally more conducive to relaxation because clients feel more anonymous; it's hard to relax when your personal trainer is watching you and you are the center of attention. In rare cases, people experience something called *relaxation anxiety* when trying to relax. This may involve discomfort with "letting go" and a fear of losing control. If your clients experience relaxation anxiety, they may have more success controlling stress with exercise than relaxation. Tell them to forget the relaxation practice if it does no good.

Cognitive Restructuring

When we can't do much to change the source of stress, we often change the way we view the problem, making the problem seem smaller and less stressful. Changing the way you think about something is called *cognitive restructuring*.

You have probably used cognitive restructuring many times, even if you never used that term. Have you ever felt like you had too much to do in too little time? Maybe you felt overwhelmed, like you could never do it all. These thoughts may have even triggered a stress response: rapid heart rate, nervousness, muscle tension, and so forth.

If you used cognitive restructuring, you calmed yourself and used positive self-talk to change the way the problem looked. You might have said something like, "I've felt like this before, and somehow I got all the work done. I'll just try to relax and focus on one thing at a time, spending more time on the most important things. I'll do the best I can, and it won't help if I get stressed out."

Although most clients are unfamiliar with the term *cognitive restructuring,* most will know what you mean when you describe self-talk as the way you talk to yourself inside your mind. Self-talk includes phrases, pictures, images, snatches of songs, and even complete sentences that you say to yourself. It runs the gamut from "I can't believe it's Thursday already!" and "The chocolate one looks good," to more emotionally laden images such as being buried in work, and phrases like, "I can't handle this," "This job is killing me," and "I'll never make it through this day." Clients may have thoughts like, "I don't have time to exercise today," or "It won't hurt if I just skip this one class," that lead them to cancel their exercise plans.

Negative self-talk often precedes a decision not to exercise as planned. Negative self-talk is usually associated with feelings of conflict and stress. As a fitness professional you can encourage clients to become aware of negative self-talk regarding physical activity, and examine the underlying beliefs that may cause these negative thoughts. You can also help clients replace negative statements with more productive and positive ones. Positive self-talk can reduce feelings of stress and help clients stick to their exercise programs. Anticipating negative self-talk and having alternative responses in place prepares clients for those occasions when they may try to talk themselves out of exercising.

Encourage clients to tune in to their self-talk, especially if it prompts them to not exercise. Self-talk can be hard to hear at first. Instruct them to pay special attention to thoughts that cause stress. This self-talk often makes mountains out of molehills, or focuses on real mountains in an unproductive worrying fashion. Ask clients with a history of exercise dropout to record negative self-talk and come up with common excuses for skipping exercise.

Give clients a week or two to write down negative self-talk about participation in physical activity. Then look at the list together. Which statements reflect real problems that need to be addressed, and which tend to be excuses? Sometimes it's hard to tell the difference. If clients say they are real problems, assume they are real problems, to begin with. Try creative problem solving for the real problems.

Then take a look at the excuses. Is there a pattern? What are the common themes? Ask clients about possible misconceptions that may lead to some of their negative self-talk. Our daily thoughts and actions

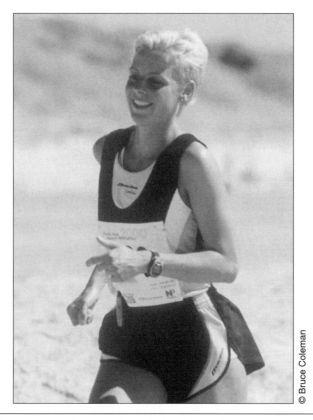

You can help your clients turn negative self-talk into positive action.

are powered by our underlying values and beliefs. Many of these are subconscious. Some clients are perfectionists and subconsciously feel like failures if their attempts are not perfect, and if they can't be perfect, they may as well not try. For example, if they don't have two hours for a complete workout, they won't work out at all. And, of course, they never get two hours.

Other excuse lists reflect an underlying belief that exercise is a waste of time and that other things are much more important. The list may reflect a subconscious belief that it is selfish to take time to exercise. Some clients seem to believe it is even wrong to have fun! These beliefs often look less powerful in the light of day and you can help clients rephrase these beliefs so that they support healthful behavior. For example, instead of believing, "Exercise is a waste of time; I have more important things to do," help your client believe that her health is a priority, and that regular exercise is vital for maintaining the good health she needs to do the "important things." Strengthen the exercise pros, and reduce the exercise cons. As you and your clients review their exercise excuse lists, encourage them to rephrase the negative self-talk into more productive (and accurate) statements.

The following list of common excuses, rephrased to promote fitness success, provides examples of how clients might rephrase negative self-talk. Do any of these phrases sound familiar? Clients may also wish to use the positive statements as an internal cheerleader to help them stick to their exercise programs.

Old: I'm too tired to work out today.

New: I'm just trying to convince myself not to exercise. But I'm going to exercise even though I feel tired, and I know I'll feel great after my workout.

Old: I'm much too busy to exercise today. I'll do it tomorrow.

New: I am really busy today, but I'm always busy. Tomorrow is not going to be much different. I'm still going to take my lunch hour to get to the gym. The exercise will give me energy and help me get more done this afternoon.

Old: It won't hurt if I just skip one day.

New: I use this excuse too often. One day turns into one month and then one year. Exercising today will help me feel great and will reinforce my commitment to staying active.

Old: This exercise program is a waste of time. I've got more important things to do.

New: I need regular exercise to stay healthy and manage stress. What's more important than my health? Staying healthy is just as important as my work, and I must make time each day to take care of myself so that I stay healthy and can work effectively.

Old: People may think I am shirking my responsibilities if I go to my noon exercise class. I'll look more responsible if I work through my lunch hour.

New: Health. Family. Work. Those are my priorities, in that order. I've made a commitment to my exercise class and I will go as planned. Responsible workers take care of their health.

Old: I'm too old for this. It's not doing me any good and I look silly.

New: Exercise is important at every age. In fact, exercise will slow the aging process. I need this exercise as much as anyone, and I'm starting to see more people my age exercising. I must be a trendsetter!

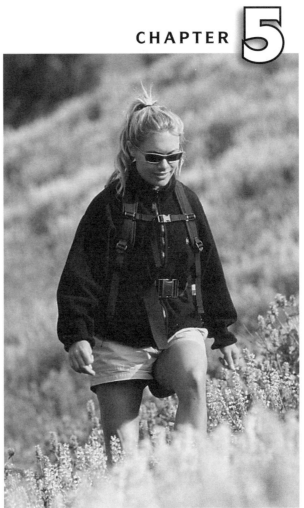

CHAPTER 5

© Bruce Coleman

Fostering Positive Exercise Experiences

Most health and fitness professionals agree that a big part of their job is fostering positive exercise experiences. It doesn't take a rocket scientist to figure out that people who enjoy working out (or at least feel good afterward) are more likely to come back for more. Whether your clients are brand new to exercise, weekend warriors, or regular fitness buffs, you are more likely to see them again if they experience positive feelings during their work with you. Personal trainers and other health and fitness professionals often spend a great deal of time crafting physiologically ideal training programs while neglecting to match the program to their clients' personal activity preferences. This chapter discusses ideas for helping clients maximize the psychological benefits of their exercise programs. The emotional rewards of physical activity reinforce exercise program adherence for everyone engaging in an exercise program.

For people participating in an exercise program, the question is not whether they will skip a few exercise sessions or drop out temporarily, but how they will deal with an episode of relapse or inactivity. Research suggests that helping people anticipate and cope with barriers to exercise enhances long-term exercise adherence (Marlatt and George 1998). You can also help your clients visualize a return to exercise after a lapse of several sessions or more. You can help clients understand that an exercise program is not an all or nothing proposition, but an opportunity to do the best they can when they find themselves in difficult situations.

The factors that motivate people to begin an exercise program appear to be different from the factors that reinforce continuing participation (Rothman 2000). People begin an exercise program because they believe regular physical activity will produce certain benefits. But they continue exercising because they actually see those (or other) benefits. This chapter presents ideas on how to help your clients see signs of progress that will reinforce their commitment to their exercise programs. Seeing progress is important for clients in action and maintenance stages.

The remainder of this chapter focuses on ideas to enhance adherence for clients in the maintenance stage. People who have been exercising regularly for at least six months have a good chance of remaining physically active. Yet this group still faces many challenges to lifelong exercise adherence. And although they may participate in some type of regular physical activity, they may still drop out of your program; therefore, they may need incentives to continue with you.

Maximizing the Psychological Benefits of Exercise

Most fitness professionals have personal experience with the psychological benefits of exercise. Most of us work in this field because of these benefits! We have had many positive exercise experiences and appreciate the way a good workout helps us feel mentally energized yet physically relaxed at the same time. We have seen ourselves and others reduce anxiety, stress, and depression with regular physical activity. We have watched people change their lives by participating in sport and other physical activity. One of the most effective ways we can enhance exercise adherence is to help our clients experience the positive emotional benefits of regular physical activity.

What Are the Psychological Benefits of Regular Physical Activity?

Studies have shown that regular exercise is associated with several important psychological benefits, including the following.

Exercise Promotes a Positive Mood

Many people report that they feel great after a good workout. To a psychologist, feeling great signifies a positive mood. A positive mood encompasses feelings of satisfaction, along with feeling happy, good, or great. People often feel energized after exercise, and have a more positive outlook on life. A positive mood may also reflect feelings of relaxation and stress reduction that commonly occur with exercise. People often say feelings of alertness combined with feelings of relaxation improve their ability to concentrate and focus. Studies have found improvements in mood after a wide variety of exercise intensities, with many different kinds of physical activity, and in almost every conceivable type of population: men, women, children, young, old, and across a wide range of fitness abilities (Brehm 2000b).

Exercise Reduces Feelings of Stress

Exercise is one of the best stress reduction techniques around, and leads to immediate and long-term results. Many people say they feel more relaxed after a single workout. Some also find that they are more relaxed when they work out regularly.

People experience stress in many different ways. Some report physical symptoms, such as muscle tension and stomachaches. Others become emotionally upset: feeling overwhelmed, pressured, or out of control. Regular physical activity helps to reduce both physical and emotional stress symptoms. Many people find that exercise helps reduce the severity of stress-related illnesses from headaches to irritable bowel disorders.

Especially important is that many people report feeling less angry and irritable when they exercise regularly. Anger is the stress factor most strongly associated with harmful health effects, such as increased risk of hypertension and heart disease (Williams and Williams 1998).

How Does It Work?

Researchers have long been intrigued by the notion of the "exercise high." Initially, positive feelings were thought to occur only with exercise of relatively high intensities or long durations. We now know that people experience positive feelings with almost every kind of exercise. And researchers now believe that exercise may lead to positive feelings for many different reasons. Here are some of the ways in which exercise may reduce feelings of stress and promote a positive mood (Brehm 1998).

- Biochemical changes in the brain: Researchers believe several different chemicals may be responsible, including endorphins, and several neurotransmitters, including serotonin and norepinephrine. The concentration of many neurochemicals changes with physical activity, but we do not yet know what types of exercise cause which changes.

- Changes in nervous system activity: The fight-or-flight response, a state of physical and psychological arousal, is associated with acute stress. Research has shown that this response is often reduced after physical exercise. It is as though regular exercise of moderate intensity provides a dress rehearsal for stress, training the body to respond with lowered physical arousal to all forms of stress, including emotional strain. Studies linking regular exercise with lower levels of arousal in response to emotional stress suggest that changes in nervous system activity may be at least partly responsible (Steptoe, Kearsley, and Walters 1993). Changes in neural response go along with biochemical changes in the central nervous system.

- Relaxed muscles: Some studies have found a decrease in electrical activity in the muscles after exercise, indicating that muscles are more relaxed (deVries, Wiswell, Bulbulian, and Moritani 1981). When your body feels physically relaxed, your mind feels more relaxed as well.

- Changes in brain wave activity: Rhythmic exercises such as walking, running, rowing, and swimming increase alpha-wave activity in the brain. Alpha waves are associated with a calm mental state, such as the one observed during meditation.

- Cognitive effects: Exercise may lead to beneficial changes in psychological state by affecting people's perceptions and thoughts. For example, exercise may provide a distraction from difficult problems. Participation in regular physical activity may give people a sense of accomplishment, self-confidence, or control, which are all powerful stress reducers. Many exercise professionals have observed that some people enjoy exercise because they feel that their activities have purpose or meaning (Morgan 2000). Exercise may lead to improvements in body image and fitness, which make people feel better. Physical activity may be perceived as fun, and as famous children's author, Dr. Seuss, once wrote, "Fun is good."

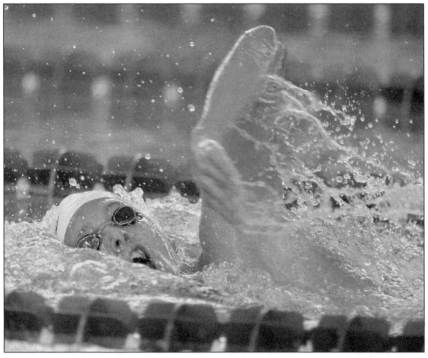

Swimming is one relaxing, rhythmic activity that both improves fitness and promotes a calm mental state.

Exercise Improves Sleep Quality

Many people report that they sleep better when they exercise regularly. Studies have found that people with moderate sleep complaints are most likely to experience improved sleep quality after participating in a program of regular exercise (King, Oman, Brassington et al. 1997; Youngstedt 1997). Typical improvements include falling asleep more quickly, longer periods of deep sleep, and feeling more refreshed in the morning.

Exercise may improve sleep quality in many ways. Because stress, anxiety, and depression can interfere with sleep quality, exercise may improve sleep in some people simply by reducing these emotional health problems. Exercise may also improve sleep through its effects on body temperature regulation (Murphy and Campbell 1997). Outdoor exercise, which provides light therapy on top of physical activity, may provide extra sleep benefits (Youngstedt 1997). Exercise also appears to have beneficial effects on sleep stage patterns, increasing the time spent in deep restorative sleep (Gambelunghe et al. 2001).

Good sleep quality improves resistance to stress-related illness and immune function. A good night's sleep helps you start the day feeling invigorated and refreshed. Good sleep habits reduce feelings of stress and improve psychological outlook. Adequate sleep allows you to experience the full energizing effect of regular physical activity.

Exercise Improves Self-Confidence and Body Image

Many people experience improved self-confidence and a better body image after several weeks of regular exercise. These improvements may even come without apparent weight loss or improvements in body composition. How can this be? Perhaps as people improve their fitness and feel stronger, their concepts of their bodies change, even though not much change occurs on the outside. After all, body image refers to the way we perceive our bodies and judge our physical attractiveness. This often has little to do with reality.

Exercise is most likely to have a positive effect on body image when people notice and value the changes that occur as a result of their exercise program. People often report feeling better about their bodies when they perceive improvements in health, fitness, or emotional well-being (Stoll and Alfermann 2002). People coping with health problems are especially likely to experience improved self-concept and body image when exercise helps them feel better and more energetic (Hurley, Mitchell, and Walsh 2003).

Unfortunately, the exercise effect on self-concept and body image is not always positive. Exercise sometimes leads to or reinforces a negative self-concept. This is most likely to occur when participation in physical activity reinforces or increases existing disparities between people's ideals of physical attractiveness and their perceptions of their appearance. This occurs most often in adolescents and young adults who value an unrealistically thin (often the case for women) or muscular (often the case for men) physique (DiBartolo and Shaffer 2002). The fitness center environment can feed into a negative body image if people feel they fall short of the fitness ideals modeled by the instructors and other clients. These negative experiences have been associated with reduced adherence to exercise (DiBartolo and Shaffer 2002).

Because most of the factors that affect a person's self-concept and body image are outside of your control, you are most likely to help people improve these variables by doing everything you can to provide positive exercise experiences. Create a friendly atmosphere that welcomes all body types. Set an example yourself, accepting yourself the way you are even as you strive to improve your fitness.

Ask clients about their reasons for exercising. Positive reasons, such as wanting to manage stress, have more energy, have fun, or improve health are associated with a better body image. Negative reasons, such as wanting to achieve a very low weight or improve appearance, are more commonly associated with negative body image and poorer exercise adherence (DiBartolo and Shaffer 2002). Suggest positive reasons for exercise as much as possible.

Exercise Reduces Feelings of Depression

Depression is characterized by a negative mood and feelings of hopelessness. All people feel depressed from time to time. A person is clinically depressed when symptoms persist for a relatively long time or when symptoms become so severe that they interfere with daily life.

Researchers have found that exercise improves mood, thus alleviating one of the most troublesome symptoms of depression. Exercise appears to be most effective when performed regularly. People with mild to moderate depression experience the greatest reductions in depression, compared to people who are not depressed or those who are severely depressed. Several studies have found that regular exercise is comparable in effectiveness to other treatments, such as medication and therapy for mild to moderate depression (Martinsen and Morgan 1997). Exercise is often used in conjunction with these other treatments.

Exercise Reduces Feelings of Anxiety

Anxiety refers to feelings of worry, self-doubt, and fearful uncertainty about the future. Researchers have studied the effect of exercise on both trait and state anxiety. *Trait anxiety* refers to the quality of anxiety as a stable personality trait; a person with high trait anxiety feels anxious much of the time. *State anxiety,* however, is situational. Most people experience temporary feelings of anxiety in certain situations, such as during a certification exam or other performance evaluation. Anxiety is a common component of stress and a frequent complaint of many clients.

Exercise has positive effects on both trait and state anxiety (Raglin 1997). While physical activity seems to reduce trait and state anxiety for both highly anxious and non-anxious people, those who experience the most anxiety often see the greatest improvements.

Exercise As Therapy: What Is Your Role?

While it is appropriate for fitness professionals to promote the psychological benefits of exercise, make sure you do not slip into the role of psychotherapist. When clients complain about stress, you can lend a sympathetic ear. You might also discuss with them how exercise might help reduce these feelings. But when clients tell you that stress, anxiety, anger, or depression is a significant force in their lives, or is interfering with their ability to function, suggest that they seek professional psychological guidance. No particular sign will signal that you should make a referral. But if you sense that emotional health issues are causing a problem for your client, ask how serious the problems are. If they interfere with daily activities, then suggest that they seek help. When you sense clients are beginning to lean too heavily on you or are relying on you to hold them together, encourage them to talk to a doctor, counselor, or therapist.

Using Psychological Benefits to Enhance Motivation and Adherence

You know that exercise provides enormous psychological benefits. Now how do you get this information, and more important, the experience of these benefits, across to your clients? How can you help your clients experience that exercise high, or that postworkout relaxation? You probably already accomplish this to some extent. You help your clients connect with psychological benefits when you ask them what they most enjoy doing, and then work these activities into your recommendations. You also help clients connect with psychological benefits when you have fun teaching a class or share your enthusiasm with a client. Maybe you remark on how great you feel after a good workout. Here are a few more ideas for helping your clients maximize the psychological benefits of exercise.

Encourage Clients to Include Emotional Balance in Their Health and Fitness Goals

Many people, especially those new to exercise, think *body* when they think *exercise*. Even fitness professionals tend to focus on the physical improvements gained through regular exercise. We use fitness assessments to measure aerobic capacity, flexibility, muscle strength, and body composition.

Educate your clients about the importance of emotional health when you discuss health and fitness goals together. Many of your clients may be concerned about stress, anxiety, and depression, but not realize that reducing these feelings is an appropriate fitness goal. Help them understand that achieving emotional balance is as appropriate as achieving a healthy weight or reducing the risk of heart disease. (In fact, reducing stress may help with weight control and reduce the risk of heart disease!) Urge them to cultivate a lifestyle that protects emotional health. Engaging in adequate self-care, including regular physical activity, is vital for emotional balance (Brehm 1998).

Ask about stress during your very first session. Include a question about stress levels on your initial assessment. For example, you might ask, "How much are you bothered by feelings of stress?" Use a scale of one to five, with one associated with "very little" and five "very much." Your client's answer to this simple question can lead to a discussion of the stress reduction benefits of exercise.

Success Story
The Power of Positive Reinforcement

Owen was assistant manager of a large fitness center in the Midwest where he also worked as a personal trainer. He shared the following account. "In my six years of personal training experience, I have found that the majority of people start exercising to lose weight, but the ones who continue exercising do so because exercise helps them feel great. I try to maximize the exercise–feel good connection as much as I can.

"At our first meeting I always ask clients about stress level when discussing health concerns and fitness goals. I rarely encounter a person who has no problem with stress. Myself included! When I ask about activity preferences, I encourage people to think creatively, and I do what I can to help them put together a program they feel excited about.

"I am still surprised at the changes I see in people. I have known clients who used exercise to cope with a difficult job or with relationship problems. Taking charge of their exercise programs seemed to help them take charge of their problems as well.

"I envision our fitness center as an emotional health oasis. People come here to recharge, refresh, and revitalize. Sure, people also exercise to lose weight or to improve appearance and health in other ways. But exercise benefits in these areas may not become apparent for weeks or even months. However, each exercise session can have an immediate emotional payback. People can get rid of their anger, irritation, and stress, and walk out feeling better. I think this is what keeps a majority of my clients coming back month after month and year after year."

Recommend Activities Clients Will Find Rewarding

Be a good listener, and encourage clients to think creatively. What activities have they found enjoyable in the past? What activities appeal most to them? Some people swear they hate to exercise. Ask them what they hate the least. Have they ever felt good *after* exercise?

As you help clients brainstorm activity preferences, consider the following.

- Outdoor activities: Sunlight and fresh air are therapeutic, especially for people who spend most of their time indoors. Consider walking, hiking, bicycling, or skating. If there's snow, recommend Nordic or alpine skiing, snowshoeing, or sledding, if appropriate. Outdoor activities can be fun, and feel more like play than exercise.

- Social support: Is there a family member or friend your client would like to exercise with? Social support improves exercise adherence, and many people find that talking as they walk is great therapy, or at least a diversion that helps pass the time. Does your client enjoy group exercise? What are the group exercise options in your area?

- Time alone: Some people need a break from other people and find that break in exercise. They may enjoy a solitary workout or being alone in a crowd.

- Time for creative thinking: Repetitive exercise modes such as walking, exercise machines, snowshoeing, hiking, bicycling, and swimming can provide quiet time to think creatively.

- Activities requiring concentration: Some people enjoy competitive sports that require total concentration, such as tennis, squash, and basketball. Outdoor adventure activities such as rock climbing and white water kayaking also require concentration. This type of concentration forces problems out of your mind and gives your brain a break from worrying.

- Competition: Similarly, many people enjoy some level of competition, whether it's a friendly recreational golf group or a highly competitive sports contest. Competition motivates clients to train, and it provides a great diversion from life's stress, unless of course the competition itself creates too much anxiety and stress! Highly competitive activities may be counterproductive for people reporting problems with stress or anxiety. Find out about the opportunities for competition in your area. Many masters programs exist for various sports. If none exist, start one at your fitness center.

- Vigorous exercise: Healthy, fairly fit people often find that vigorous activity provides greater stress relief than exercise of a more moderate intensity. Urge these clients to step up the pace. Suggest interval training to pump up the metabolic rate, or working out longer over the weekend or whenever they have the time. Caution: Be sure vigorous exercise is appropriate for your client before recommending it.

- Mind–body activities: In disciplines such as yoga and tai chi, the participant strives for emotional balance through activity. These activities, which are becoming popular and more widely available, are usually appropriate for a wide range of fitness levels and ages, and many people find them a nice change of pace.

- Rhythmic breathing: Rhythmic breathing is often a component of mind–body activities and may be partly responsible for a relaxed and meditative mental state. Other activities such as swimming and running may also involve rhythmic breathing.

- Recreational activities: Just about any activity perceived as enjoyable has psychological benefits. Nothing beats having a good time or building a sense of accomplishment. Of course, as you help clients select activities, you will want to find activities that help clients move toward all of their fitness goals. For example, if they want to go bowling, they may wish to choose additional activities for the cardiovascular system.

- Activities with a purpose: Many exercise professionals have observed that people who successfully incorporate physical activity into their lives year after year, decade after decade, do so because the chosen activity has a purpose. People may walk or bike for transportation or garden in order to have beautiful flowers or fresh vegetables.

- Meaning: Perhaps the greatest psychological benefit of physical activity is finding meaning—in the best case, meaning in life, but meaning in the activity is also beneficial. For example, many people enjoy connecting with nature while hiking. Others train for physical activities that involve fundraising for meaningful charities. Physical activity may provide a vehicle for strengthening a relationship with a family member or friend. Mind–body activities may involve a search for emotional balance and philosophical understanding.

Measure Improvements in Mood and Energy Level

If clients consciously try to see psychological benefits in their exercise programs, they are more likely to experience them and to figure out what kinds of exercise deliver the greatest psychological benefits. Sometimes just knowing they might experience these benefits helps clients see changes. If you work with a client on a regular basis, you might consider using a questionnaire that measures improvement in mood either after a workout or after several weeks of regular exercise (see figure 5.1) (Annesi 1996; Gauvin and Rejeski 1993). To measure the immediate effects of exercise, ask the client to fill out the questionnaire before and after exercise, then see if anything changes. To analyze long-term changes, compare questionnaires administered several weeks apart.

While many people experience measurable improvement in mood and energy level after exercise, not everyone does, and many people do not experience it after each workout. Don't be too disappointed if you do not find change. The psychological benefits may come later in the day, or they may build over time. People experiencing significant anxiety or

Instructions: Please use the following scale to indicate the extent to which each word below describes *how you feel at this moment in time.* Record your responses by filling in the appropriate circle next to each word.

0 = Do Not Feel (DNF)
1 = Feel Slightly
2 = Feel Moderately
3 = Feel Strongly
4 = Feel Very Strongly (FVS)

	DNF 0 1 2 3 4 FVS		DNF 0 1 2 3 4 FVS
1. Refreshed	o o o o o	7. Happy	o o o o o
2. Calm	o o o o o	8. Tired	o o o o o
3. Fatigued	o o o o o	9. Revived	o o o o o
4. Enthusiastic	o o o o o	10. Peaceful	o o o o o
5. Relaxed	o o o o o	11. Worn out	o o o o o
6. Energetic	o o o o o	12. Upbeat	o o o o o

Figure 5.1 Scoring for the Exercise-Induced Feeling Inventory (EFI)
The EFI consists of four distinct subscales. Subscale scores are obtained by summing or averaging the numerical values chosen for the adjectives within a particular subscale. The four subscales include (1) Positive Engagement (items 4, 7, and 12); (2) Revitalization (items 1, 6, and 9); (3) Tranquility (items 2, 5, and 10); and (4) Physical Exhaustion (items 3, 8, and 11).

Reprinted, by permission, from L. Gauvin and W.J. Rejeski, 1993, "The exercise-induced feeling inventory: Development and initial validation," *Journal of Sport and Exercise Psychology* 15(4): 403-423.

depression may not see benefits for several weeks. Therefore, although it is reasonable to look for psychological benefits, be careful not to oversell them or build up unrealistic expectations.

Asking clients if they experience psychological changes with exercise can also help you determine if the exercise program is *not* working. For example, if clients complain that exercise feels too difficult or that they feel exhausted after exercise rather than invigorated, you may need to modify the exercise program. Try decreasing the exercise intensity or the amount of exercise your client performs. Some clients have a very low tolerance for vigorous exercise. They interpret a rapid heart rate as panic or tired muscles as exhaustion. This may change over time, but these clients will probably drop out before they adjust their perceptions. Start them extra easy, even though you know they could do more. Other clients, especially those new to exercise, may have trouble regulating exercise intensity. They may start out at a sprint and tire quickly.

Q&A

Q Do people who hate to exercise ever learn to enjoy it?

A Yes, many people who say they hate exercise eventually come around to enjoying it or at least appreciating its multiple benefits. Much of the change comes as people learn to think about exercise in new ways. Some begin to exercise regularly to cope with a health condition, such as hypertension or type 2 diabetes. Their doctors may have urged them to become more active, or they may have read something that convinced them that exercise would be a good idea. Some people begin to appreciate exercise after they try a new activity and find that they enjoy it. Others try exercising in new ways that make exercise more tolerable. For example, people who hate exercise because they find it boring sometimes enjoy exercising while talking with a friend. Or they find another diversion, such as watching television, reading, or listening to music, while exercising that helps the time pass more quickly. Some people learn to hate exercise because prior experiences have been painful or embarrassing. Try to get your clients to tell you what they dislike about exercise, and then use this information to design a program that is more likely to be successful. Many people, for example, begin exercising at an intensity that leads to discomfort or even injury. Recommend comfortable activities and intensities.

Do clients need clarification on regulating exercise intensity? Many clients new to exercise find target heart rates very confusing. In addition, the target heart rates you calculate may not fit a given individual, especially if you use predicted maximal heart rate in your calculations. Consider teaching your clients to regulate exercise intensity by using rate of perceived exertion (Borg 1982). Or, simply advise them to exercise at an intensity that feels a little challenging, but not too hard. Some health and fitness professionals counsel people to use the talk–sing test. Because singing requires a slower breathing rate, people should have enough breath to talk during exercise, but should work hard enough that singing is difficult.

Helping Clients Anticipate and Plan for Disruption

Your clients can come up with a million reasons to skip a workout. You have probably heard them all by now and used some of them yourself! Exercising is a difficult behavior to maintain because it takes a great deal of time and energy. And in truth, some days it is nearly impossible to fit it in. Help clients acknowledge this, and anticipate and plan for disruption.

Anticipating and planning for disruption can lead to several positive results (Marlatt and George 1998). First, anticipating disruptions and planning for them allow clients to work around interruptions and stick to their programs, even if they must modify them. Second, when clients anticipate disruption they are not surprised when they must miss a workout. Instead of thinking, *This is it, the end of my exercise program,* they understand that disruptions are a part of life and that they must go with the flow but figure out ways to resume regular exercise.

At your first session with a new client you probably asked him about previous experience with exercise programs. You may have discussed what he sees as the barriers to exercise participation. Perhaps you came up with solutions to these early barriers, or at least ways to work around them. This type of discussion lays the groundwork for further discussion of possible problems that might arise and gives your client practice in solving problems.

In the previous chapter we discussed using counterconditioning and stimulus control to cope with barriers to exercise. Both techniques anticipate problems that might interfere with exercise participation. Counterconditioning modifies a person's response to the problem, and stimulus control modifies the problem itself. No matter what you call your problem solving techniques, they all boil down to asking your clients what might interfere with their exercise programs and doing your best to come up with workable solutions to potential problems.

Learning From Relapse and From Success

Relapse means returning to behavior patterns, such as being sedentary or overeating, that you have attempted to change. People who have started an exercise program relapse if they quit exercising for an extended period of time. If your client drops out of activities for a week or two because of travel, illness, or other disruptions, it is not a relapse if they resume their activities after that week or two. The danger, of course, is that a short period of inactivity can lead to an indefinite relapse. The best way to help clients anticipate disruption is to ask them to think about difficulties that have kept them from exercising and about previous experiences with relapse. Encourage clients to learn from these experiences to understand the emotional and physical factors that have caused lapses in their exercise program participation. Once they acknowledge these factors, you can help them plan ways to deal with them if they occur again. Similarly, you can learn from past successes. These experiences are easier to talk about and will give your clients positive feelings.

Fitness professionals may behave as though relapse behavior means one thing: failure, both on the part of the fitness professional and on the part of the client. Because failure may cause embarrassment and shame, we avoid talking about it. However, this thinking is unproductive and leads to missed opportunities. It blocks creative problem solving, hurts self-esteem, and undermines future success. While it is natural to be disappointed when we fail to achieve important goals, we must help ourselves and our clients view behavior change as a lifelong process that requires patience, understanding, and compassion. You can help your clients learn from their relapses, and this learning can increase the likelihood of success in future behavior change efforts. Help your clients see prior failures as learning opportunities, rather than indicators of limited potential or personal weakness.

You may have asked clients what worked and what didn't work when you met them at their first session. These early discussions are usually superficial and brief. When you have time, help clients explore relapse experiences and success experiences in more depth. Ask about these experiences. Be a good listener, and work with clients to figure out how to use this knowledge to improve their chances of success.

While each client is different, common themes in exercise relapse often emerge. Some of the most common problems include the following:

- Plans to exercise were not specific enough. People often resolve to become more active, but they fail to nail down a specific plan of action. In fact, the need for a specific program may have brought clients to you! People who work with a fitness professional to design specific exercise programs that match their health concerns, fitness goals, and exercise preferences are much more likely to still be exercising six months later than someone who simply resolves to start exercising.

- Goals were not realistic. We discussed this problem at length in chapter 3. Lofty goals sound great and are very motivational, but when progress is slow, people tend to become discouraged and give up.

- The exercise program was too demanding. Many people quit if the exercise feels too hard or takes too much time. If people have quit for either of these reasons, be sure they perceive their current exercise program as achievable.

- A disruption in routine threw off the exercise schedule. Once clients set an exercise program in motion, they often rely on the force of habit to keep it going. Anything that disrupts their routine can lead to relapse. In reality, most people's lives are filled with disruption: changes in schedule, unforeseen events, visitors, travel, holidays, injury, and illness, to name a few. Help clients learn from past disruptions and use their problem solving skills to plan for future disruptions. What will they do when they get sick? Travel? Must stay home with the children on a snow day? What will they do when it starts getting dark early? Accommodation for disruption must be built into every exercise program.

- Negative moods reduced the motivation to stick to an exercise program. Feelings of stress and depression reduce the motivation to change a habit. Exercising may not seem important any more in the face of negative feelings. How will clients cope with these feelings when they rise again? Check the section called Managing Stress and Negative Emotions in chapter 4 for help with this.

Coach Clients to Imagine a Return After Relapse

Encourage clients to admit that sometime, perhaps soon, something will force them to temporarily abandon their exercise plans. How might this happen? What will it feel like? And how will they get back into exercising regularly?

The bottom line is that clients must realize that skipping a class should not be construed as a failure, and when this happens, the best thing is to think about how they will get to their next exercise session. Clients must also learn not to let feelings of failure get in the way of their commitment to their exercise program.

Measuring Progress and Finding Improvement

People are more likely to continue exercising when they have concrete evidence that they are earning returns on their exercise investment. Your clients probably began an exercise program because they believed it would yield certain benefits. You have coached them to expect realistic benefits. How do you help them see that the program is delivering as promised? How do you help them experience the improvements in fitness and health that will reinforce their commitment to regular physical activity?

Many fitness professionals know that measuring the improvements from an exercise program can be a double-edged sword. When improvement occurs, clients are happy and motivated. But if they don't see improvement, clients become discouraged, sometimes discouraged enough to quit exercising. If the exercise does no good, why bother?

Clients are more likely to progress toward their goals if you have helped them establish both process and product goals. Your clients reach process goals simply doing what they have decided to do, such as attend three workouts a week or walk a certain distance. Your clients may not yet have seen physical improvements, especially if it is the very beginning of an exercise program, but they have achieved goals. And in truth, process goals are the most important, because regular exercise eventually will lead to physiological and psychological improvement. Your client's exercise log attests to the successful completion of these process goals.

Some fitness centers use computer programs that compile members' workouts and provide extensive feedback on an assortment of workout variables. Evidence suggests that this extensive record keeping and feedback is motivational for many people (Annesi 1998). If you do not have access to the required equipment, help clients record workouts in another way. Many fitness centers provide cards for recording workouts. Over time, clients see that they are lifting more weight, performing more reps, or staying on a cardio machine longer.

What kind of fitness product goals might your clients achieve? These will depend on the exercise program you have recommended. Most clients will see progress in the amount of exercise they can do. In six to eight weeks they may see that they can complete more repetitions of a weight training exercise or move up to using a greater resistance. They may increase their work level on a piece of cardiovascular training equipment, or they may stay on the machine longer. Point out this progress to your clients and acknowledge their improvement. Clients starting at low fitness levels will experience the greatest improvement rates early

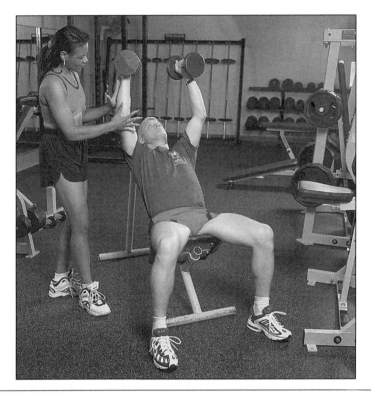

Seemingly small changes—the ability to lift more weight or to increase sets and reps—can be very motivating for your clients.

in their programs. Take advantage of this fact to motivate your clients to continue exercising.

What about other fitness measures? You will only find improvement in the fitness variables your clients are training, so focus your observations on these and don't test areas that are not likely to improve. If you have worked with people for many years, you probably know the types of improvement you are likely to find and when you are likely to find them. Here are a few of the most common indicators of fitness improvement:

- Emotional health indicators: We mention these first, because they are the most likely to show short-term improvement. These were discussed at the beginning of this chapter.

- Resting heart rate: Many trainers ask their clients to measure resting heart rate, either first thing in the morning or before falling asleep at night. Be sure clients understand the variables that can affect resting heart rate, such as illness, stress, caffeine, alcohol, menstrual cycle, and so forth. Give specific instructions on how to take a resting heart rate. Clients new to exercise often experience a decrease in resting heart rate after a few months of exercise.

- Heart rate during a given submaximal workload: Clients performing aerobic exercise are also likely to experience a decrease in exercise heart rate for exercise performed at a standard workload on a piece of equipment that reproduces the type of exercise training the client is performing. People who walk regularly on a treadmill may see a decrease in exercise heart rate when walking at a given workload, but may not see a drop in exercise heart rate when pedaling a cycle ergometer. If you measure submaximal heart rate periodically, remember that you must be very exacting with your workload administration. "Level 5" may vary from one machine to the next. Be sure that the submaximal load or loads are identical each time you test your client.

- Muscle strength and endurance: Gains in muscle strength and endurance occur fairly quickly during the first few months of an exercise program. Most adult exercisers are happy to see their reps and weights go up on their workout cards. Many personal trainers forego strength tests in favor of these improvements. If you give a strength test, be sure that it will not cause muscle soreness or injury.

- Walking test: Measuring fitness improvement with a timed walking test usually yields positive results if clients have been walking for several weeks as part of their exercise programs.

- Flexibility: Flexibility is slow to improve, but you may see progress after several weeks of exercise that includes regular stretching.

- Balance: Balance measurements show the most improvement for adults participating in some sort of balance training program, which is increasingly popular with older adults.

- Skill level: Clients participating in an activity that improves a skill, such as rock climbing, tennis, or golf, will be pleased to see improvements in motor skills. Work with these clients to establish realistic ways to gauge skill improvement in a given activity.

- Medical indicators, such as resting blood pressure, blood lipid levels, blood sugar levels, or bone density: If any of these are the focus of your clients' exercise programs, discuss the types of progress they are likely to see. Your clients' health care providers should establish regular intervals for measuring these indicators. Many factors, including diet or changes in weight, can affect these indicators, so take this into consideration when evaluating exercise results.

- Body weight: Body weight is easily measured, but is a poor indicator of body composition changes. Body weight may stay the same even after body composition has changed, or it may fluctuate by several pounds with changes in hydration. Nevertheless, clients on a weight reduction program who are more than a few pounds overweight will probably see a decrease in weight. Urge them to work for slow weight loss that is likely to stay off. Good luck, and do what you can to reduce the obsession with the bathroom scale.

- Body size: Clients who are only slightly overweight may not see much change in scale weight, but body composition changes (fat loss with an increase in muscle mass) may lead to a change in body size. Many people are happy when a waistband on a skirt or pair of pants fits more loosely. Therefore, many trainers encourage clients to watch for changes in the way their clothes fit.

- Body composition: If you measure body composition, be sure your measurements are as accurate and reliable as possible. Inform clients about the measurement errors inherent in these devices. Because changes in body composition may take months to register on a body composition test, show your clients other ways to see that their exercise programs are yielding positive results.

Q&A

Q Should you give every client a fitness assessment? And how often should these assessments be given?

A Many people find fitness assessments intimidating, so I do not recommend them for everyone. The people who need exercise the most often receive poor scores on fitness assessments, which can be demoralizing. In addition, if a fitness assessment is required for beginning an exercise program, many people see this as one more reason to postpone beginning an exercise program. Why increase the barriers to participation in regular physical activity? If we make beginning an exercise program as easy and painless as possible, we are likely to attract more people. If you or your fitness center offer a fitness assessment program, we suggest making it optional. People with an exercise history may want to take a battery of fitness tests. For these people, the tests provide interesting information and serve as a benchmark for improvement. Finding improvements in fitness is motivational, so if you retest, wait for at least three months of good attendance. Meanwhile, be sure clients find progress in other ways.

Reinforcing Commitment in Experienced Exercisers

Fitness professionals often work with clients in the maintenance stage of readiness, people who have been exercising regularly for six months or longer. Even though these people are likely to remain physically active, they may or may not choose to continue working with you. Unless they believe that your program meets their needs, they may start looking for variety or a change. How do you meet the needs of this diverse group?

When you work with a new client who is already an experienced exerciser, your approach is not so different from the way you start with someone new to exercise. You listen carefully as you help the client establish fitness goals and as you discuss health concerns. Why has this person decided to meet with a trainer? A client who is already active usually has specific questions and goals. Do your best to answer questions and give the sophisticated advice these clients may be looking for.

Never take your long-term clients and members for granted. Experienced exercisers may change their exercise programs when they begin to get bored with the same old activities, or because they feel they have reached a plateau in fitness improvements. You may be able to entice these people to remain interested in your advice and your programs by offering them new exercise horizons. Consider these ways of providing variety and renewing interest in your programs:

- Encourage clients to learn a new sport or activity.
- Encourage clients to consider participating in masters competitions for the sport of their choice.
- Help clients set new goals. Perhaps they would enjoy training for a special event, such as a marathon or bikeathon. Periodized training might provide the training stimulus and the variety these clients are looking for.
- Provide continuing education on exercise benefits and ways to remain active throughout the seasons and the years.
- Provide incentives for remaining with you: special recognition or discounts. Offer special opportunities, such as a free fitness checkup or personal training session. Celebrate the anniversary of the day they started working with you.
- Encourage clients to expand the psychological benefits of their exercise programs. Teach them to use visualization and mindful awareness to increase these benefits.

- If feasible, encourage people to increase their activity volume and intensity to see greater fitness improvements.
- Do what you can to help your clients find meaning and to connect with others through the exercise experience. Make the exercise program rewarding and meaningful.

Experienced exercisers do drop out of exercise programs, and even quit exercising. While minor disruptions are unlikely to throw them off course, the larger problems that occur in every life may keep them away from exercise for a while. These challenges include becoming a parent, experiencing significant difficulties at work or at home, health problems, or moving to a new location. Work with your clients who face these issues. Help them adjust their exercise expectations and figure out new ways to continue to be active.

Q&A

Q I know regular exercise is a good thing, but some people come to the fitness center where I work almost every single day and they work out for more than two hours each time. When does commitment to exercise turn into compulsive exercising? Should I be concerned about these people?

A Unless one of these people is a personal training client or student of yours or they bother other users, there is not much you can do. Some exercise regularly to manage stress and hold themselves together. As long is this does not harm them or anyone else, it is not up to you to intervene. Some people use excessive exercise as part of their recovery from a more serious addiction, such as an alcohol problem or eating disorder. Some people *do* become obsessive and compulsive about their exercise programs. This obsession becomes noticeable when exercisers won't stop exercising even when continuing causes damage. For example, while it is normal to want to continue exercising through an overuse injury, the correct response is to take time off if necessary or to find an alternative type of exercise that will allow the injury to heal. Clients who exercise compulsively will continue to engage in exercise even when that activity makes an illness or injury worse. If you have a client who matches this description, then by all means voice your concern. Help him work out ways to exercise that will allow the injury to heal, and refer him to a counselor if he needs help changing his exercise routine because of an exercise dependency.

CHAPTER 6

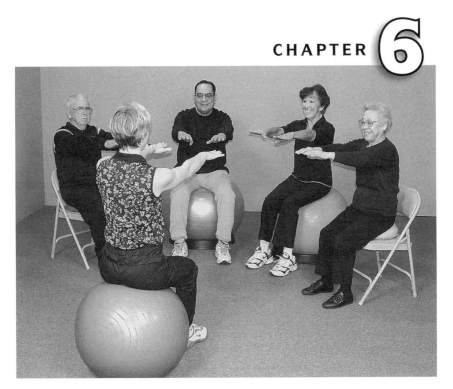

Working With the Clinical Population: Focus on Ability

You know from your work that each person is a unique individual. No matter where you work, whether in a community recreation program, a health club, a worksite fitness setting, a rehabilitation setting, or in people's homes, you are bound to encounter a wide range of health concerns and fitness goals. You may have noticed by now that even apparently healthy people sometimes have concerns about future health problems, perhaps about conditions that run in their families. You have probably seen your share of knee problems and low-back pain. Perhaps you have worked with adults already diagnosed with hypertension or type 2 diabetes.

If current health trends continue, we are likely to see more fitness professionals working in clinical settings and more people with health problems in fitness settings. As the number of older adults climbs dramatically, and as the prevalence of obesity remains high or grows higher, we are likely to see a steady rise in the number of people with chronic health problems (Booth and Chakravarthy 2002). These problems include type 2 diabetes, hypertension, heart disease, arthritis, and osteoporosis.

Not only are more people chronically ill, but more people with chronic illnesses are advised by their health care providers to become more active. Research continues to support the idea that exercise is good medicine. The American College of Sports Medicine (1997) has published guidelines for prescribing exercises to counteract 40 separate medical conditions. In some cases, regular exercise helps to treat symptoms. In others, exercise improves functional ability and enhances quality of life. Many people with chronic illness exercise in order to preserve their freedom and independence.

Accessible Exercise: Limited for People With Special Needs

Research shows that exercise offers immeasurable physical and psychological health benefits for almost everyone, including most people with chronic illnesses and disabilities. Exercise can substantially improve physical function and quality of life. But the barriers to physical activity for people with special needs are often enormous. Here are a few of the most problematic:

- Accessibility: People with limited mobility may have difficulty finding opportunities to move. If they cannot walk, they may only be able to exercise with special equipment such as weights and exercise machines, or in a pool. Access to these may require special transportation and facilities that are wheelchair accessible.

- Qualified fitness professionals: Few fitness professionals are trained to recommend exercise to people with special needs. Working with special populations requires additional education and training not readily available to most fitness professionals.

- Medical clearance: Many physicians are reluctant to recommend exercise for people with chronic health problems because they don't know what to recommend and because they fear that injury could lead to litigation.

- Financial resources: Medical insurance reimbursement for exercise expenses is extremely limited. Patients may be reimbursed for physical therapy, but for only a very short time if you consider that most patients need to engage in lifelong activity. Because job opportunities are limited for many people with chronic health problems, their financial resources may be limited. This can make exercise classes, personal trainers, and fitness center memberships unaffordable.

For more information on the need for accessible exercise, and on physical activity opportunities for people with special needs, log on to The National Center on Physical Activity and Disability at www.ncpad.org.

Exercise specialists work with people from the clinical population in a variety of settings. These include hospitals, hospital-affiliated fitness centers, and various types of rehabilitation centers. Some work in health club settings that allow rehab patients access to their facilities at certain hours, or for special programs run in conjunction with physical therapy or other rehabilitation groups. Some personal trainers work in traditional fitness settings but with clients who have been referred by their physicians. The clinical setting can even include a client's home.

The largest market segment for personal trainers continues to be apparently healthy adults with general fitness goals. However, the fastest growing segment includes clients with special needs, such as those who have just finished some sort of rehab program, or clients with special health issues and goals. The *clinical population* in this chapter refers to people who have sought treatment for medical conditions, or who are under medical supervision for a health problem. You may work with them in their rehabilitation programs or as they shift from a medically supervised rehabilitation program to community- or home-based programs. Some people in the clinical population recover significantly and return to the activities they enjoyed before they became patients. Others have progressive diseases that worsen over time; they may exercise to slow loss of functional ability and to improve quality of life (Smith 2000).

This chapter focuses on exercise adherence in clinical populations. While much of the information presented in this book can be applied to health and fitness professionals working in a clinical setting and to those who work with people who have health problems, this chapter addresses some of the issues specific to working with clinical populations. This chapter first discusses the challenges of a medical setting and the importance of teamwork in this setting. Most exercise specialists in clinical settings work as part of a medical team that includes physical therapists, physicians, nurses, social workers, and other health care providers. This chapter takes a look at how teamwork affects your work with patients and clients, and your strategies to motivate them to make their health and recovery a priority.

Next, the chapter examines factors that enhance adherence in clinical populations. Your ability to develop good working relationships with your clients is one of the most important. The first step in connecting with people from the clinical population is to understand their health concerns and their journeys through the labyrinths of biomedicine. These journeys often leave people feeling hopeless and helpless, and one of your most important jobs is to help clients change their self-concepts from "disabled patients" to "regular exercisers."

People seeking your help in the clinical setting may or may not be ready to undertake an exercise rehabilitation program. You might think that because they have been told to exercise and are coming to you for advice, they are at least in the preparation stage. This is not necessarily the case; their health history may have pushed them into your office and they may not understand the commitment you will ask them to make. Assessing your patients' or clients' readiness to incorporate exercise into their lives will help you tailor your advice so it will be as helpful as possible. This chapter discusses how to use this information to help people shape exercise goals and programs that facilitate recovery and improve quality of life.

Clients and patients in the clinical setting often have low exercise self-efficacy. This chapter explores why and presents strategies to improve this important variable. It also looks at the barriers to exercise that people from the clinical population face and presents ideas for maximizing exercise adherence despite difficulties.

The Clinical Setting: When Clients Are Patients

One of the main differences between health club clients and a clinical population is that your clients enter the clinical setting as patients. In order to understand how this role interferes with exercise adherence, think back to the last time you visited a hospital as a "client," either as a patient yourself or as you helped a hospitalized friend or family member.

How does it feel to be a patient? Some people report positive hospital experiences, especially when the health problem is not perceived to be serious, and when recovery is expected to be rapid. They appreciate the medical expertise and intervention, and feel supported and helped by the medical staff. But many people who are hospitalized for a health problem report feeling worried or even frightened about their health, especially when the health problem is seen as threatening (Kabat-Zinn 1990). Many report feeling frustrated by and angry with medical bureaucracy, where many different professionals treat different parts of them. People who have been hospitalized often report feeling unimportant and powerless, wishing providers were more available, and listened more to their concerns. The hospital environment can feel noisy, cold, and indifferent, as overworked hospital staff struggle to keep up with the piles of forms that must be completed. And it can be depressing to be around a lot of very sick people.

Traditional medicine, known in the field of sociology as biomedicine, has been remarkably successful in treating many health problems. This success has come from medicine's focus on biological systems and biochemistry, and medicine's ability to study and understand the biological processes of disease.

However, this specialized focus often leaves patients feeling dissatisfied with their medical treatments because it omits many factors important to health and healing processes. Although physicians may thoroughly understand the bypass operations they recommend, they may overlook the lifestyle that led to the artery disease they are now trying to repair. In some cases, biomedicine can worsen conditions that cause disease in the first place, conditions such as depression, isolation, and loneliness (Ornish 1998). Physicians have been spending less time with each patient over the past several years. Many patients report significant levels of stress, depression, and other forms of emotional and physical distress.

Many people emerge from encounters with biomedical systems hungry for connection and understanding, and with a strong longing for holistic therapies that treat the whole person, not just the disease. Health and fitness professionals are in a position to capitalize on growing consumer demand for holistic medical therapies. Beginning an exercise program is the perfect antidote to the helpless, hopeless feelings that being a medical patient can prompt. Instead of focusing on the disease, health and fitness professionals can maximize the positive force of exercise by focusing on the whole person, the active person working to regain strength and ability, and to improve quality of life.

Creating a holistic approach in your practice can enrich your life and add meaning to your career path. Cultivating a holistic approach is not difficult if you simply imagine how you would like to be treated if you were one of your clients. What would you look for in a health and fitness professional? You would probably prefer an exercise specialist with good medical knowledge who communicates an attitude of respect and caring. You will have the greatest success motivating people in the clinical setting when you try to understand and connect with your patients or clients, as described in chapter 1.

"Anything that promotes a sense of isolation often leads to illness and suffering. Anything that promotes a sense of . . . connection and community is healing."

—*Dean Ornish, from* Love and Survival: 8 Pathways to Intimacy and Health

Teamwork in the Clinical Setting

One of the biggest differences between working in a fitness center and in a clinical setting is the importance of your role as medical team member. While in a traditional fitness center you may work with other professionals, such as other trainers, instructors, and so forth to coordinate your work, in a clinical setting your teamwork tends to be more complex. Physicians and other health care providers count on you to understand patients' exercise prescriptions and exercise limitations. And patients often ask you to help them interpret medical instructions from their physicians, dieticians, and other therapists.

This chapter assumes you have the training, certifications, and medical expertise required for the clinical work you do. But to work effectively in the clinical setting, it helps to have a strong medical team behind your efforts to motivate clients and help guide them toward dedication to lifelong exercise. Patients are also more likely to follow "doctor's orders," in this case to exercise regularly, when the medical team works together to provide a consistent message. People want reassurance that your exercise recommendations are an important and integral part of their treatment plan (Smith 2000).

Think for a moment about your medical team. What about the team works well? Fitness professionals working in the clinical setting have described factors that contribute to an effective team, not to mention a better work environment for all team members (Mutrie 1999). Here are some of the most important factors that contribute to good teamwork.

- Common philosophy: Teams work best when members share a similar philosophy, mission statement, and vision of how their team should function, and what sort of experience the person receiving care will have. In the clinical setting, quality patient care and respect for the patient should be the focus.

- Understanding of and respect for each other's work: Each person understands clearly which role each team member plays and respects the importance of that role in the treatment process. Each person acts autonomously in certain areas, but knows when to consult other team members.

- Clear understanding of communication channels: Medical staff can be extremely busy, so communication between members should be efficient and effective. Busy people often prefer a written note or e-mail to a phone call or meeting. Is this the case on your team? If you need to talk, when are the best times to call? Do the physicians want to talk to you directly, or do you work through a nurse? If you are new to a medical team, be sure to find out the best way to get in touch with other team members.

- Good organization: Good organization reduces frustration and wasted time, and supports efficient work. Procedures are clear. Equipment is clean and in good repair. Quality of care improves when workers are not distracted by the frustration and pressure of a disorganized workplace.

- Problems are dealt with as they arise: Problems are a fact of life. A good team has established systems and uses them to deal with problems they encounter in their work. Good communication channels enhance effective problem solving.

Success Story
Networks of Support

Heather works in a physical therapy clinic associated with a large hospital. She had this to say about teamwork: "I primarily work with the other physical therapists in our clinic. While a large group of physicians refers patients to our program, we are pretty autonomous. The docs send the patients in to us, and we do our thing.

"I still see teamwork as being very important to the quality of care we give the patients, and to the quality of my job. We have a good team here in the rehab unit. We meet regularly, have regular trainings, and everyone has a great attitude. We try to create an atmosphere of fun and good humor.

"We don't have a great deal of contact with most of the physicians, although they do come in sometimes to talk about a certain patient, or check someone's records. But when we have questions, we know how to get information to one another, and whom to contact. And I really feel supported by the physicians and other providers. They let us know that our work is important. We have very good adherence rates for the patients who go through our program, and I think a lot of it is due to the fact that we all give the patients the same message: You have to go through rehab and develop a regular exercise program.

"Why did I move from the sports clinic to a rehab setting? The work just feels more meaningful to me here. The stakes are higher, but the work is rewarding. Many of our patients come to us in pretty bad shape, but after a few months they start putting their lives back together in a whole new way. I often get to know their families and friends. I feel like my work here really makes a difference to a lot of people."

Factors That Affect Adherence in Clinical Populations

Many studies have looked at adherence in people who begin an exercise program to rehabilitate an injury or to treat illness. When health problems arise and health care providers advise patients that exercise is important, many patients are motivated to begin exercising. The exercise pros quickly outweigh the exercise cons. In addition, people in a rehabilitation situation may have contact with fitness professionals and other therapists that helps keep them going. Ideally, if exercise seems to provide therapeutic results, people will continue to exercise in order to maximize the benefits of regular physical activity.

But as with any group beginning an exercise program, some will stay and some will go. Here are some of the other factors related to adherence in the clinical population.

History of Regular Physical Activity

People who were fairly active before illness or injury are likely to believe in the importance of exercise and want to return as soon as possible to the activities they enjoy. Those who followed a structured exercise program may still have the wherewithal for a repeat performance. They've done it before, so they know they can do it again, although perhaps in a different form. They have moved through the stages of change in terms of exercise readiness, and may come to you more prepared to begin a new exercise program.

Belief in the Efficacy of the Exercise Recommendations

People who believe their exercise programs will have a positive effect are more motivated to follow exercise recommendations. Do everything you can do to increase your client's belief in the efficacy of your recommendations. As mentioned before, consistent endorsement by the medical team, especially the client's physician, helps to reinforce your words. If your client seems to need more information about the efficacy of exercise for his problem, give him articles and handouts that confirm the information you give him. As he starts to recover and make progress, point out that the exercise is making him stronger.

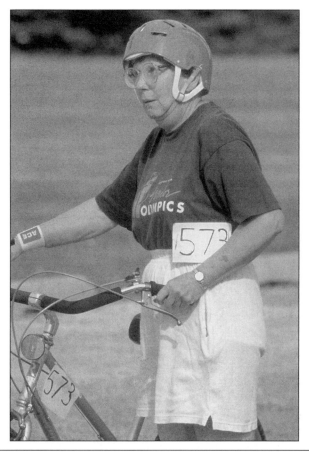

If your clients and patients *believe* that they can make physical activity a regular part of their lives, they are more likely to do so.

Thoughts and Beliefs About Health Problems

Beliefs in the efficacy of the exercise recommendations are intertwined with people's beliefs about their illnesses or injuries. People who believe that they are vulnerable to future health problems may feel more motivated to keep up with their exercise programs if they feel exercise may reduce the threat of future problems. You can help people with chronic health problems understand the nature of their illnesses or injuries, and how exercise therapy slows the loss of function or improves quality of life. People recovering from a heart attack, for example, need to learn about the types of heart disease they have and their prognosis for recovery. Explain how regular physical activity plays into this prognosis. Ideally, you want clients to believe that they have power over the progression of their health problems or at least the quality of their lives.

Q&A

Q I have just begun working with a woman who is recovering from breast cancer. She told me her illness was pretty serious and that although she feels better now, there is a good chance of the cancer recurring. I didn't know what to say when she told me this; what should I say to a client who may not get better or may even die?

A These are difficult situations, especially for fitness professionals accustomed to dealing only with apparently healthy people and who have had little personal contact with serious illnesses. I applaud your willingness to work with this client. Many people recovering from or living with cancer choose to exercise to recover from the side effects of their cancer treatments, for example, surgery, chemotherapy or radiation therapy, and to improve their quality of life. There is no "right" thing to say when you learn that a client faces a possibly terminal illness. A cancer survivor once remarked that there is only one thing all people with cancer would like to hear: "It's all been a mistake. You don't really have cancer and you're going to be fine." Because we are not in a position to deliver this remark, we can only acknowledge the client's words and the difficulty of the situation.

If you are meeting with the client for the first time, allow her to share as much as she wishes. Some people want to talk about their experiences and others do not. If you are still getting to know this client, respect her limits and carry on as you would with any other client. Knowing that she may eventually die does not really affect your work with her today. Keep your focus on the present and on improving quality of life, just as you would were her condition less serious. While her risk of dying may be higher than yours at this moment, we are all at risk. The mortality rate for humans is 100 percent. And who knows, she may still outlive you. You may wish to learn more about living with a cancer diagnosis so that you feel more comfortable working with her and eventually with other clients, family, and friends who may face a life-threatening illness. A good source for information on living with cancer may be found at the American Cancer Society's Web site, www.cancer.org. Information on working with people who may have a terminal illness may be found at the Web site for Hospice Net, www.hospicenet.org.

Understanding Instructions

People who drop out of their exercise rehabilitation programs sometimes say they quit because they didn't understand the exercise recommendations. Health and fitness professionals may find this a lame excuse; we would likely go back to the therapist and ask questions! But imagine a patient unfamiliar with the rehab environment, perhaps someone feeling sick, weak, or depressed. Unclear instructions might lead to frustration or a fear of doing something wrong that could cause further injury. When patients feel powerless, they may feel like giving up because they do not have the energy to contact the therapist to clarify the instructions.

Research on adherence to medical treatment plans suggests that our communications, as providers, often miss their mark (Clark and Becker 1998; Ley 1976). Studies suggest that patients remember only about half of the instructions received after the first five minutes of an explanation. Instructions and explanations are best remembered when information is categorized and simplified as much as possible. Patients have the best recall of information presented at the beginning of a session, so start with the most important instructions and explanations first.

A lack of understanding is most likely to occur when you see patients briefly or for very few sessions. Take your anticipated time with each patient into account as you plan your training sessions. Be sure you explain everything very clearly and check frequently to make sure that the person understands what you are saying. People struggling to cope with health problems may be somewhat disoriented and have a hard time concentrating on your instructions. Certain medications may interfere with learning, as well. Be sure all instructions are written down, and keep your recommendations as simple as possible if your patient seems to have trouble understanding.

Contact With Rehabilitation Professionals

Longer contact with rehabilitation professionals, at least during the initial stage of treatment, improves exercise adherence in many cases. More time with the exercise specialist might mean a better understanding of the exercise recommendations, a stronger belief in the efficacy of the treatment, and perhaps the establishment of an exercise habit. However, extended contact with exercise specialists must be convenient and affordable. When this contact becomes too inconvenient or expensive, it becomes a barrier to exercise.

Plans for the Future

People who are driven to recover lost function or to slow disease progression are more likely to translate this drive into action, in this case, adherence to an exercise program. Many therapists have observed how people with potentially debilitating and painful conditions will persist in therapy because they must get better in order to return to work or an unfinished project, or to take care of a spouse, relative, friend, or even a pet. Trainers who work with athletes have observed how injured athletes determined to overcome illness or injury in order to be ready for future competition can make truly remarkable progress. The will to recover can fuel a person's passion for life and commitment to exercise rehabilitation. When you work with people from the clinical population, talk to them about their hopes for the future. Link these goals to regular physical activity.

Perceived Social Support

When people perceive that others are there for them, helping them and cheering them on, adherence improves. Interestingly, *perceived* social support is more important than the actual number of people providing logistical social support, although logistical support is extremely important, too. Perceived social support has more to do with feeling like you care for and are cared for by other people (Ornish 1998).

The strongest forms of social support come from caring family, friends, and community. But your clients may also perceive you and the rest of the medical team to be supportive as well. You have probably seen how different patients or clients have very different perceptions of you and the support you offer. Some are open and trusting, and if you work together for an extended time, they may treat you as an adopted family member, even if they do not know you very well. They may joke with you, show you pictures of their families and pets, and tell everyone else how great you are. This perceived connection provides comfort and connection and should be encouraged, in the context of your professional behavior, of course. This connection helps people relax and cope with stress and illness, and therefore has great healing power.

At the other extreme, you may have patients or clients who are cold and aloof. They may appear angry, depressed, or withdrawn. While you offer them the same support you offer every client, they do not perceive you to be support. Unless they receive effective support elsewhere, these patients or clients are generally less likely to be successful in sticking to their exercise programs.

Q&A

Q What can you do when patients or clients have no support?

A Sometimes you may see patients or clients who appear to have no support. No friends or family come along or seem to visit. However, sometimes support is in the wings, but you just don't see it. If you ask, you may find that relatives live far away and don't have a chance to visit often. But they may call regularly and provide support via telephone or e-mail. Some people have neighbors who stop in and help from time to time. Perhaps charitable groups include this person in their work. People from religious or community groups may stop by with a basket of fruit and stay for a visit. These activities help a person feel supported and cared for. If your patient or client has none of these connections in his life, do you have ideas for creating them? Maybe the social workers in your team have ideas. You and your medical team can try to provide positive emotional support when these people are in your care. The most difficult patients or clients are those who appear to be alone in the world and are also irritable, angry, or depressed. They may not be much fun to be around, and they may seem unapproachable to those who want to help. If you have a patient or client who fits this description, do what you can to be supportive. Spend a few extra minutes talking to him. Ask him about the book he is reading, the pictures on his table, the handmade blanket on his lap. Try to get him involved in activities available to him. Get the social workers and other therapists on your team to help you. You and other staff members can make a difference in this person's life and create a sense of caring that might help him work through his negative feelings.

Logistical Support

Logistical support helps clients stick to their exercise programs. People may help with transportation, household chores, or child care. Close friends and family members may attend exercise counseling sessions with your client to help interpret instructions or to provide emotional support. When this is the case, incorporate the helper as much as possible if you think this help will be beneficial.

Comfort of the Clinical Environment

Comfort means different things to different people. In general, people are comfortable when they feel emotionally welcome and at home. The office staff checks them in with courtesy, they have a comfortable place to wait, they don't wait too long, and the therapists are pleasant. Of course the physical environment also affects comfort. The medical environment should exude cheerfulness, as well as cleanliness.

Scheduling Convenience

Exercise is a difficult habit to establish. Why give people an excuse, such as inconvenience, to drop out? Work with your medical team to devise solutions to the scheduling problems your patients or clients encounter.

Discomfort or Pain During Activity

Discomfort and pain are common barriers to exercise in the clinical population (Dunlap and Barry 1999). Many people new to exercise drop out when exercise is too intense or uncomfortable. People who come to you with health problems may not be very fit. If this is the case, they may tire quickly during physical activity. They may find even relatively low levels of exertion uncomfortable. Now add pain to this picture. Imagine being not only new to exercise, but coping with pain. The last thing you would want to do is cause yourself more pain. Pain often creates feelings of fear (of worsening pain or injury), which in turn create more pain.

Try to devise exercise recommendations that produce the least amount of discomfort or pain possible. Even if the exercise program lacks the intensity ideal for producing substantial therapeutic results, your patient or client will reap some benefit from beginning an exercise program. You can up the intensity later after an exercise habit has been established and after exercise tolerance improves.

When pain is problematic for your patients or clients, encourage or help them work with their health care providers to better address pain management. Many patients become frustrated when pain control is inadequate. Finding adequate pain control may take time and a period of trial and error, experimenting with various medications and other pain control measures.

What if activity is painful? Check back with your patient's provider to be sure you understand activity limitations. In some cases, mild pain can be tolerated for the sake of rehabilitation and later pain reduction. But unless you are a physical therapist and are trained to deal with patients who must work with pain, pain is a signal to stop and evaluate your exercise recommendations to ensure that they are safe.

Patients and clients appreciate advice on how to differentiate between harmful and harmless pain. People with arthritis, for example, should be taught how to discriminate between "good" pain, such as normal muscle fatigue, and "bad" pain, such as sharp joint pain (Nelson et al. 2002).

Stage Theory in the Clinical Population

The strength of a stage-based approach to exercise program design is that it is client focused. Getting a general sense of how people feel about starting or changing their exercise programs will help guide your recommendations. You will be more successful in your work when you try to match the treatment to the client, help clients become psychologically ready for exercise, and work with them to increase their commitment to an exercise program (Mutrie 1999).

During your first session with a patient or client, you want to find out how ready she is to take on an exercise program. In many cases, as when a physician prescribes exercise, we assume that people are ready to jump into action and get started. You have probably noticed that this is not always the case. As you talk to your patient or client about her health concerns, recent health problems, and exercise history, you can ask her how she feels about starting a new program. Your discussion will give you a sense of her readiness to begin and her level of exercise self-efficacy.

When your patients or clients are reluctant to exercise or do not seem to believe that an exercise program is necessary, you need to discuss their beliefs about their health and the importance of an exercise program. Previously sedentary people respond better to a counseling approach that gives them time to express themselves and their concerns, than to jumping right into a fitness assessment and exercise (Mutrie 1999). Listen carefully to your patients' or clients' concerns, and ask questions that help people explore solutions to their problems. Correct misunderstandings about their health conditions. Address fears. Provide educational materials to help them understand why exercise is important.

Ask physicians to emphasize the importance of the exercise prescription. A health problem is often a great motivator, and a doctor's admonition to exercise can quickly move people from precontemplation into contemplation and preparation. The balance of exercise pros and cons shifts dramatically. For clients who seem stuck in precontemplation or contemplation, motivational interviewing techniques (see chapter 3) may be helpful.

Q&A

Q At the center where I work, our patients start their rehab routine the day they come in. We are expected to get them moving right away, and with our heavy schedule, I don't see myself spending an hour discussing exercise pros and cons with each patient! How do you fit all of this counseling into a clinical setting?

A There are many ways to talk with your patients. If your patients are participating in an exercise routine, talk to them while they exercise. Ask questions while they ride the cycle ergometer, or walk on the treadmill or track. Walking programs can be a great opportunity to talk with patients individually or in small groups. If you work with groups of patients, put patients of similar readiness together so you can talk with several people at once. They can also talk with each other and share their concerns as they exercise. You can pair more advanced and committed exercisers with people new to (and reluctant to begin) an exercise program. Do you lead a group warm-up? Cool-down? Stretching session? You can initiate discussions during these sessions once patients know the routine. Take advantage of your medical team. Who else is counseling your patients? Can the dietitians put in a strong plug for exercise? You can do the same for diet. What information do they get from the physicians, nurses, and other providers? Social workers and occupational therapists? Keep in mind, too, that time at the clinic spent talking and connecting with your patients is time well spent. Getting patients to sign on to a lifelong exercise program is an important goal, just as important as getting them through the exercise session they are to perform on a given day.

Motivational Goals and Behavior Change Skills

As health and fitness professionals we have therapeutic goals for our patients and clients. These reflect not only people's health problems, but also how much time we have to work with them. We recommend exercise to increase muscle strength, joint stability, and cardiovascular endurance. These phrases may not be meaningful to many of your patients or clients, however. When you begin working with new people, ask them to describe what they would like to achieve through an exercise program. Therapeutic goals will be more motivational if you can help people set goals that are meaningful to them.

Research shows that the most common exercise program goals for clients and patients in the clinical setting are to feel better physically, feel better psychologically, and prevent or slow further decline (Mutrie 1999). The more you can establish the link between physical activity and these goals, the better your chance of enhancing exercise adherence.

As always, goals must be specific for each client or patient. What does feeling better physically mean? How could exercise help increase strength or reduce pain? Encourage your patients and clients from the clinical population to look for the psychological benefits that might come from an exercise program. Include these benefits as goals for the exercise program. Explain to people that physical activity may help them feel more energetic and positive, less stressed, and stronger physically and emotionally. Exercise can help people with health problems feel more able, and you can help to keep the focus on enlarging the repertoire of what people *can* do, rather than focusing on what has been lost. Research suggests that as self-efficacy in the exercise arena improves, people also feel more in control of other facets of disease management. For example, dietary and medication measures may improve in people with diabetes (Vasterling, Sementilli, and Burish 1988).

What is your patient's prognosis? Can exercise increase the likelihood of full recovery? Enhance partial recovery? Delay decline? In what ways? Whether someone's goals are full recovery or slowing the loss of function, explain how exercise can affect these goals. What kinds of exercise are best and how will you measure progress toward these goals? For example, people recovering from a heart attack will want to reduce risk of another heart attack, or slow the process of artery disease. Progress might be measured by improved aerobic capacity and cardiac function, better blood lipid control, weight loss, or reduced blood pressure. People with osteoporosis may exercise to slow the loss of bone mass, increase joint strength and balance, and reduce the risk of falling. Progress might be a favorable result on a bone density test, the ability to lift more weight during a given exercise, or better scores on a balance test.

Frail patients and clients may set exercise goals focused on the tasks of daily living. Some want to get strong enough to leave the hospital or rehab center and go home. Those already at home may want to be able to maintain independent living as long as possible. Link their exercise programs to the abilities they need, such as the strength to use the stairs, carry groceries, and carry out housekeeping tasks.

As you discuss goals with your patients or clients, focus on quality of life. What really matters most to them now? What would they *like* to be able to do? Spend time with family and friends? Return to a job or volunteer position? What will it take to get them there? What sign posts along the way will indicate that they are making progress? Harnessing the power of hope will increase exercise adherence and improve quality of life.

When the Goal Is Weight Loss

Many health and fitness professionals may find themselves working with people whose physicians have told them to lose weight. Even a relatively small weight loss can improve blood sugar regulation, blood pressure, and blood lipids, and ease stress on vulnerable joints. Many people find it difficult to lose weight, and find it even more difficult to keep the weight off.

When you help people set weight loss goals, be sure to include process goals along with your product goal (weight loss). Goals can take the form of exercise program adherence, for example, walking a certain number of miles per day or week. Exercise provides the best foundation for a weight loss program because in addition to burning calories, it improves mood. Unfortunately, most people focus on dietary restriction when trying to lose weight, which can lead to feelings of deprivation and stress. Granted, people must restrict calorie intake to lose weight; exercise alone will rarely do the trick. But dietary restriction is easier to bear when your mood is lifted by physical activity.

Once you and your client have a good set of goals and have designed an appropriate exercise program, talk about the importance of sticking to the program. Teach the behavior change skills described in chapter 4. These work equally well with the clinical population (Clark and Becker 1998; Duncan and Pozehl 2002). These include the following:

- Self-monitor. Encourage people to keep track of their workouts on a calendar or exercise log. You can monitor these records as well.

- Monitor progress. As you monitor people's records, keep track of signs of progress toward their goals. These might be as simple as completing a certain number of exercise sessions, or they might be measures of progress on a fitness test. Monitor psychological progress in terms of improvement in mood and energy level.

- Anticipate and solve problems. Use stimulus control, counter-conditioning, and other problem solving techniques to plan ahead for problems that could interfere with exercise adherence. Identify triggers for skipping an exercise session, and major disruptions such as travel, holidays, out-of-town guests, and so forth, just as you would with any other client. Help people dream up effective ways to deal with upcoming events that could disrupt their exercise routines.

- Teach ways to manage stress and cope with negative emotions. Negative emotions are a leading cause of exercise dropout in the clinical population, just as they are in the apparently healthy population. The healthy pleasures (see page 84) and mindful awareness (see page 85) exercises, and the cognitive restructuring information from chapter 4 may help people improve stress management skills.

Building Exercise Self-Efficacy

Building exercise self-efficacy in the clinical population is the same in principle as building exercise self-efficacy in apparently healthy people (Clark and Becker 1998). The activities may differ, of course, depending on the types of health problems you are dealing with. The following are ideas for increasing exercise self-efficacy in your patients or clients:

- Let people experience immediate success. Introduce new skills slowly, allowing people to master a few new skills at each session. You may feel that progress is very slow, but slow progress is better than confusion.

- Bring in good role models. People coping with difficult health problems are relieved when they see people like themselves exercising and making progress. Bring in people to give a pep talk that says, "If I can do it, so can you!" As you look for role models, remember to consider not only the health problem but also other factors such as age, gender, and ethnic background that will lead your patients or clients to identify with the role model. If live role models are unavailable, turn to books, articles, or videos.

- Encourage exercise partners. Exercise partners are just as powerful in the clinical setting as they are in more mainstream environments. Partners help and encourage each other, and people will do things for a partner, such as exercise, that they might not do for themselves. Partners need to be compatible with each other in terms of ability and personality, so let people choose their own partners if possible. Often spouses, other family members, and close friends will volunteer to act as exercise partners. Sometimes partners will evolve naturally out of small groups that you put together.

- Provide plenty of positive reinforcement. Positive reinforcement can take many forms. Your words of praise are important. Reinforce positive client behaviors, such as regular attendance and working correctly. Measure, record, and reward progress in all areas. Be sure to keep track of psychological improvements as well as physical improvements.

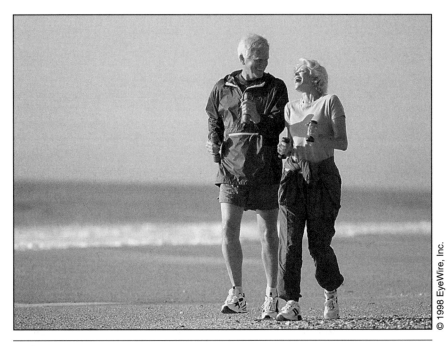

© 1998 EyeWire, Inc.

Exercise partnership is one very effective form of encouragement that may help your clients and patients stick with their programs.

- Encourage people to change counterproductive thoughts. If you work with people for several weeks or more, you may have a chance to participate in cognitive restructuring with them, either informally as you talk together, or in a more structured way using the suggestions from the Cognitive Restructuring section in chapter 4. You can encourage people to examine negative self-talk, such as "I can't do this," " I might as well give up," or "There's no point to this." Help them question unproductive thoughts and beliefs, and replace counterproductive thoughts with more positive ones.

Success Story _____
The Power of Positive Thinking

Todd, who works in the cardiac rehab unit of a large urban hospital, had this to say about the important roles attitude and self-efficacy play in exercise adherence: "In my experience, self-efficacy is the most important predictor of rehab success. You see some people who have just given up and refuse to try, even though their prognosis is no worse than most of the other patients who come out of surgery. Others have a tremendous will to recover and live full lives, even though you might think they have reason to be discouraged.

"One of the patients I will never forget is a great example of what self-efficacy can do. At the age of 84, Bud was experiencing chest pain. He was extremely healthy except for a few clogged arteries, so he ended up with a triple bypass. He had such a positive attitude about his whole medical experience, that he was a pleasure to work with. His wife told me that as they wheeled him off for his surgery, he was singing, 'Off We Go Into the Wild Blue Yonder.'

"Bypass surgery is no picnic at any age. Bud did his best to ignore the pain and discomfort, and kept his focus on getting well. He took all his rehab instructions very seriously and couldn't wait to start his walking program as soon as possible.

"You know, I think some of the reason he recovered so quickly was his strong faith in his medical team. He was always saying what a great doctor he had and how we were all doing such a good job. I think he wanted to believe that, and so he did. Of course, we all did our best to confirm his expectations!

"I wish I could take credit for his success. He got the standard cardiac rehab exercise program, and of course, with his good attitude, we all looked forward to his appearance in the rehab center and did everything we could for him. He liked to cheer up the other patients. I remember the cardiologist taking him around to visit all the other recovering bypass patients one day to show him off. The message was, 'If this 84-year-old man can recover, so can you!'

"Of course, he had everything going for him. A caring wife who made sure he took his medicine and followed the dietary instructions. She walked with him every day once he was back home. Incredible social support—there was a steady stream of visitors once he was out of the woods—big family, lots of people from his church, strong religious faith. He had a lot to live for. He said he had to get better quickly because he had two college graduations to get to.

"I wish I could capture some of his positive attitude, distill it, and hand it out to all of the other patients. I guess some people are just born lucky. But I also know Bud made a lot of conscious choices to live well and get as much out of life as possible, which for him meant giving back to others. He has been an inspiration to us all."

Overcoming Barriers to Exercise

Barriers to exercise exist in any population. However, the barriers to exercise for people with health limitations are generally greater than they are for those who are healthy. You may have to be creative as you work with your patients and clients to anticipate and deal with potential barriers. Some of the most common include the following (Dunlap and Barry 1999).

Access to Exercise

As described at the beginning of this chapter, access to exercise opportunities is limited for many people with health problems. Facilities, classes, and instructors may be inaccessible because of limitations in the physical environment or a lack of adequate financial resources or both. These problems can be difficult to solve. Examine all of the options available to your patient or client. If he will exercise at home, help him come up with a program using affordable or make-it-yourself equipment.

Depression

Depression is more prevalent in patients with severe chronic medical conditions than in those without. Some studies estimate that depression affects about 10 percent of those receiving medical treatment. Studies estimate that only about 30 to 35 percent of these cases are diagnosed and treated (Nease and Malouin 2003).

The special challenge of depression is that it often leads to feelings of lethargy and a lack of motivation to exercise or be active. Even though you tell your patients or clients that exercise will help them feel more energetic, they may not have the energy to put on their walking shoes and get out of the house. If you suspect that a patient or client is suffering from depression, point out the signs and symptoms that concern you, and suggest that she talk to her doctor. Suggest that exercise be part of the treatment plan.

Multiple Health Problems and Medication Side Effects

In addition to a person's primary medical focus, other illnesses and limitations may exist simultaneously. They may be related to the original problem, as when a person with artery disease also has type 2 diabetes. Or they may be unrelated, such as when a person who has emphysema also happens to have osteoarthritis in both knees. The more numerous and complex the health issues, the more limited the possible exercise recommendations.

People with several different health issues often feel frustrated because exercise or medical advice for one contradicts the advice for another. Help these people sort out the priorities and find activities that will work. Be sure your client's health care provider is aware of and treating all of the medical conditions.

Sometimes certain conditions, such as dizziness, are medication side effects. People often neglect to mention problematic symptoms to their physicians. Encourage people to take their concerns to their physicians. Sometimes medications can be changed or dosages adjusted to reduce problematic side effects.

Pain

Pain is associated with most medical problems. Pain is usually perceived as a warning to rest the afflicted area. Unfortunately, pain may be continuous in some medical conditions, such as many forms of arthritis. And rest and inactivity make pain worse for some conditions. Pain can also be a symptom of depression or another medical problem, such as a sleep disorder. When should someone exercise with pain, and when should a certain amount of pain be tolerated? Educate yourself about the health conditions you work with, and work closely with the medical staff on your team to be sure the pain is being controlled as well as it can be and that your exercise advice is sound.

Fear of Harm

People coping with health problems, especially those new to exercise, may feel fragile and vulnerable. Their bodies are already experiencing limitations, and they don't want to compromise their abilities further. Your clients may fear falling or suffering another heart attack. People with chronic obstructive pulmonary disease may fear becoming short of breath.

Much has been written about the importance of making exercise environments as safe as possible (Balady et al. 1998; McInnis and Balady 1999). And you will certainly do everything you can to be sure your patients or clients exercise within their prescribed recommendations and in environments suitable for their risk levels. When people voice concerns about the safety of their exercise programs, ask them what worries them about the exercises. Remind them that their physicians recommended these exercises and that they are an important part of their treatment programs. Then reassure them about the safety of their exercise programs, and emphasize that the substantial benefits to be gained from exercising far outweigh hypothetical risks. Review with people their exercise limits and the warning signs that might indicate that they should stop exercising.

Fear does not always respond to rational argument, however. Begin your fearful clients with low-intensity, gentle exercise to help them get over their fears, and to show them that they can exercise safely.

Low Exercise Self-Efficacy

People who are still reeling from their illness or injury experiences may feel powerless, hopeless, helpless, and stressed. Help to increase their self-efficacy by using the suggestions given for improving exercise self-efficacy earlier in this chapter.

The exercise environment is important for building self-efficacy. Medical fitness centers attract many people who would otherwise feel uncomfortable in an exercise environment. People who are at low fitness levels or have little experience with exercise often feel out of place in a more mainstream setting. So do people who are overweight or older. Make sure your environment is welcoming and feels physically and emotionally safe (Milner 2002). Be sure your environment and programs deliver the caring, high-quality treatment your patients or clients desire.

Low Fitness Levels and a History of Sedentary Lifestyle

Low fitness levels combined with other health limitations indicate a program of extremely low exercise volumes at low intensities. The good news is that people at low initial fitness levels are likely to see improvements from an exercise program in a relatively short time. People who have never embraced an active lifestyle may need extra education about the benefits of physical activity in order to move through the contemplation and preparation stages of exercise readiness.

Sometimes people who have never seen the need for exercise change their point of view once they see that exercise is vital to their recovery and their ability to live independent lives. Vince is the director of a rehabilitation and wellness center in a small town. His center is associated with but physically separate from the community hospital. His center is used during certain hours for physical therapy and is open as a fitness center during other hours. Many of his clients make the transition to the fitness center and its programs after completing their rehabilitation programs. He made the following observations.

"Many of our clients are older adults, and most do not have much of an exercise history. They're out of shape from their illnesses and surgeries, and starting pretty much from scratch. It's amazing to watch the progress many of them have made. We have excellent adherence, and many of our members have been with us for years. Lots of them come to us after orthopedic surgery; many have had hip and knee replacements. They see how important exercise is for recovery, and they know they'll deteriorate quickly without it. We offer a variety of personal training services, and classes in aerobics, tai chi, and balance and core stabilization. Our classes are small and our instructors are very well trained. I think our clients feel safer here than they would at a more conventional fitness center."

Because we, as health and fitness professionals, often have extended contact with people during or after the rehabilitation period, we can play a key role in motivating them and enhancing their adherence to their exercise programs. We can work as healers who confirm our clients' wholeness as we work to see them as people, not just patients. We can help people from the clinical population focus on what they can do, rather than the abilities they may have lost. We can bring a sense of normalcy, fun, and humor into peoples' lives. We can help them understand that regular physical activity is an affirmation of life, an expression of the will to live, and the desire to make the most of each day.

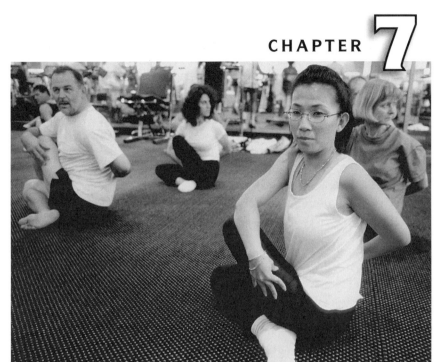

CHAPTER 7

© Sport The Library

Motivational Strategies for Group Exercise Leaders

Many fitness professionals work in group exercise settings. The information in the previous chapters provides the foundation for understanding the processes of behavior change and the many factors that influence exercise adherence for those you work with in your group exercise programs. However, motivating a group of exercisers differs in many ways from designing motivational strategies for individuals. This chapter explores ways to help you increase exercise adherence for people in group exercise settings.

Group exercise can occur in a wide variety of settings. You might teach a class in a health club, community center, or at a worksite. Most colleges and universities offer activity programs. Hospitals, nursing homes, and residential communities sometimes sponsor opportunities for group exercise. Many instructors choose to work independently, renting space and developing their own programs and classes.

Group exercise classes vary in size and structure. Two people can make a group, or perhaps you have more than a hundred people in one class. In many groups the participants actively exercise during the entire session with you. Other groups incorporate discussion and non-exercise activities into the group format. And some groups are discussion only, with participants exercising at other times. The motivational strategies you apply in your group exercise program will depend on your exercise setting and the nature of your group.

People enjoy group exercise for many reasons. Some find that they push themselves a little harder when they are part of a group. Wanting to keep up with their classmates and the instructor, they complete a few more exercise repetitions in the group than they would on their own. Many people like group exercise because they don't have to decide what to do next. (And they don't have the opportunity to decide to exercise tomorrow instead!) The teacher decides for them.

Group exercise can prevent boredom and help the exercise time pass quickly. The instructors are entertaining and the music invigorating. And the choreography and instructions keep your mind busy and your eyes off the clock. The right kind of class provides an atmosphere that is motivational, challenging, energizing, and supportive. The instructor and your fellow exercisers can motivate you to complete the workout even when you don't really feel like it.

Some people participate in group exercise to have access to a knowledgeable and helpful fitness professional who designs a safe workout, answers their questions, and provides them with educational advice. They appreciate the fact that their instructor can help them adapt the exercise to their health and fitness concerns and check to see that they are performing the exercises properly.

People in an exercise group often motivate and support each other, both inside and outside of class. Members of the group may hesitate to skip a session because they know their absence will be noticed. They may even look forward to seeing some of the other participants, which helps them attend regularly. Even though group members may only be casual acquaintances, the connection fostered by regular participation in the group exercise program helps to enhance exercise adherence.

This chapter opens with an exploration of the question: Do people have better exercise adherence when they participate in group exercise programs or when they exercise on their own? The issues raised by this question help us begin to see the factors associated with group exercise that can enhance or deter participation.

Group exercise instructors are usually interested not only in whether their participants exercise regularly, but more specifically in whether they attend the instructor's group exercise program regularly and then sign up for the next session. In most fitness businesses, numbers count. Group exercise instructors are often judged by the number of participants they draw to their classes. This chapter looks at the factors that boost adherence to group exercise programs.

The most important factor contributing to exercise adherence in group exercise settings is the quality of instruction. We explore the many variables that go into quality instruction and discuss how understanding and developing a good rapport with clients distinguishes high-quality instructors from those who merely show up.

Many of the skills you teach in a personal training setting can be taught in a group setting. We examine ways to help your participants increase exercise self-efficacy and improve behavior change skills. We also discuss the importance of the "fun factor," and present ideas for fostering positive emotional experiences in your exercise group that keep participants coming back for more.

Does Participation in Group Exercise Enhance Adherence?

Researchers have wondered whether people who exercise in a group format are more likely to stick to their exercise programs than people who exercise on their own. Not surprisingly, some research says yes (Annesi 1999; Carron et al. 1996), while other research says no (King et al. 1997; Ransdell et al. 2003). Group experience is attractive to some people for the many reasons listed previously. However, group exercise can also impose its own set of barriers that may discourage regular attendance. Here are some of the factors that affect adherence to group exercise programs.

Convenience

One of the primary reasons people stop attending group exercise programs is the extra time commitment. Not only does the exercise session itself take time, but traveling to the class location requires even more. Time is often a barrier to exercise adherence, so anything that increases the time required to exercise can deter participation.

In addition, group exercise classes must be scheduled for specific times. If a person can't get to class at a particular time, exercise may not occur. Busy people with crazy schedules often find themselves unable to get to class because "something came up." And people's schedules change, so a time that was once convenient might become difficult.

People who are considering joining a group exercise program should consider convenience. They should choose an exercise site that does not require much travel time. Do group exercise options exist at their worksite? Near their work location? Near home? On the way home? The less travel time, the better.

Check-in for class should also be fast and convenient. People should not have to wait in line to sign in or pick up towels. If people drive to the class location, parking should be convenient.

When are the group exercise classes offered? Do these times fit conveniently into the person's schedule? Many larger fitness centers offer flexibility in terms of group exercise options. Some let people come during several time slots; if people miss the 5:00 class, they are welcome to attend the 6:00 class. More flexibility means fewer excuses for missing an exercise session.

How long does the class itself last? Most people prefer classes that are an hour or less in length. While some people enjoy a longer, more thorough workout, most people say that longer classes take too much time.

Too Many Missed Classes Lead to Dropout

When people miss more than a few group exercise sessions, they become reluctant to rejoin the group. They worry that they will not know what's going on or that the instructor will be annoyed because they have missed too many classes. They may be disappointed in themselves and start thinking of themselves as failures and exercise dropouts. These negative thoughts create more stress and dampen motivation to get to class.

Some group exercise instructors try to combat this all-or-nothing thinking by discussing with their groups how to deal with attendance lapses. You can try to help your clients anticipate problems that may interfere with class attendance. In addition, you can let them know that some people need to miss several exercise sessions for various reasons, such as illness or travel. While emphasizing the importance of regular exercise and attendance, reassure them that you understand that lives can be complicated and that you will not take absences personally. Make suggestions for staying active when they can't get to class, and reinforce the importance of returning to the class as soon as possible.

Some instructors ask their participants to call or e-mail if they must miss a class. This only makes sense if people must register for your particular group and are expected to come to most sessions. In these situations, instructors often call people who have missed one or two sessions to find out if there is a problem. This gives you an opportunity to solicit feedback from your client; is something about the class not working? Maybe it is something you can fix. Checking in with absent clients also lets them know they were missed. You can reassure them that they will be able to catch up and fit right back in. Checking in helps them maintain a positive connection with you so they don't feel so bad about returning after missing a few sessions.

Body Composition

Several studies have found that people who are overweight tend to experience poorer attendance in group exercise settings than those who are not overweight and tend to prefer home-based exercise programs (King et al. 1997; Perri et al. 1997). There are probably many reasons for this. People who are overweight may feel embarrassed exercising in front of others, feeling that their bodies are being appraised and criticized by the other class participants. They may also move more slowly than others in the class, and if the class is moving at a certain tempo, they may simply be uncomfortable moving that quickly. The same thing may be true for taller people in the class. Longer or larger arms and legs take more time to move through a given range of motion.

If the extra weight is accompanied by a lower fitness level, the class pace may be more difficult for your overweight clients. Remember that people are more likely to drop out of an exercise program that feels too difficult. Intense exercise may be exhilarating for people in good shape but just feels too difficult for everyone else.

When working with overweight clients to find appropriate exercise options, ask them about their preferences. Each person is different, so don't assume every overweight person prefers a home-based exercise program. If they're interested in trying a class, suggest group options that match their interests and fitness levels and steer them toward groups you feel will be comfortable for them.

Compatibility of the Exercise Class

People will be more likely to attend a group exercise program if they feel comfortable with the group. People who see themselves as different from the other group members may be reluctant to exercise with the group. It may be uncomfortable to be the only man in an exercise class. Similarly, an older person may feel out of place in a group of people in their 20s. As stated in the previous section, it's no fun to be overweight and out of shape in a group of fit and slender athletes.

If you are a personal trainer, help your clients interested in group exercise find classes that are a good match for their fitness levels. If you are a group exercise instructor and one of your participants feels the group is not a good match, recommend a class that might work better. It's especially important that the class be appropriate for your client's fitness level.

Stress

People who feel stressed generally have poorer exercise adherence. Stress takes less of a toll on group exercise adherence, however, than on individually based exercise programs. This makes sense if you recall the information on self-control presented in chapter 4. Stress reduces an individual's self-control energy, making it harder to mobilize the energy required to stick to exercise plans. The more decisions you must make during an exercise session, the more stress reduces exercise adherence. There are too many opportunities to cut corners or to cut out exercise altogether.

The more that exercise is part of a routine, the more likely it is that a person will continue to exercise even when feeling stressed. Group exercise is nice in this way. You go to class, and once you get there, little self-control is required; the instructor and the group carry you along. Group exercise can be a good stress reducer, too. While you may continue to dwell on your problems if you work out alone, a group exercise class may provide a stronger diversion that helps to take your mind off of your problems.

Exercise Environment

People are more likely to enjoy a group exercise class if the class environment is comfortable. The temperature should not be too hot, and the air circulation should be good. The room should be clean and attractive. Limit your group to the room's capacity; overcrowding makes people uncomfortable and increases injury risk. If you use music, it should suit the group and not be too loud. People should be able to hear your instructions easily.

Quality Instruction Improves Exercise Adherence

Many of the people who decide to attend your group exercise program will already have had experience in group exercise classes. Several of them will be somewhat informed about the fitness business and have fairly high expectations for exercise instructor qualifications. Some may even ask about your certifications, education, and years of teaching experience. If they don't ask, tell them anyway! Consumers like to know they are in good hands, so don't be afraid to blow your own horn. When you introduce yourself, include a few of your most impressive qualifications. Describe your exercise science degree, your years of teaching, or your expertise in working with people who have their particular health problems. These important credentials help you gain your clients' trust and confidence.

Your class will also expect a high degree of professionalism from you. You know what that means. Simple details such as starting and ending class on time, coming well prepared for each session, dressing appropriately, and designing a well-constructed class establish your reputation as a professional instructor. Clients expect you to teach them about injury prevention, correct exercise positions and movements, and how to work at the right exercise intensity. You treat each participant with respect and an open, nonjudgmental attitude. They look to you for inspiration as a positive role model of a healthful lifestyle.

Experienced instructors develop an ability to match their class routine to their participants and to alter their plan if the class needs to go more slowly or more quickly. Good instructors watch their group carefully, gauging how the class is going and quickly modifying their plan if people have difficulty or start looking bored. Rather than watching their own reflections in the mirror, their eyes scan the crowd, giving feedback and corrections, and making decisions about what to do next.

A Motivational Leadership Style Improves Adherence

What constitutes a motivational leadership style in a group exercise setting? In general, you let your participants know you care about their fitness success and that you will do everything you can to help motivate them and give them the skills they need to reach their fitness goals. You enhance the motivation of your participants when you make them feel welcome in your group and when you let them know they are working correctly and making progress. This means giving each person a little bit of individual attention at each class. You motivate your participants to stick to their exercise programs when you help to foster positive exercise experiences. A motivational leader is a lot like a cheerleader. Your job is to get people's energy and spirits up. You want people to walk out of your class feeling great!

Research suggests that people have more positive feelings about a group exercise class when they receive more attention and encouragement from the instructor (Turner, Rejeski, and Brawley 1997). Continued personal connection and support from an instructor over time encourages exercise adherence (Castro, King, and Brassington 2001; Young and King 1997). Following are some of the things you can do to make a positive connection with your participants.

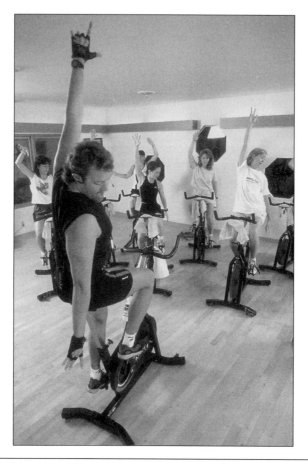

An energetic, enthusiastic instructor can keep participants coming back for more.

Give Individual Attention Using People's Names

Think of it as an opportunity to improve your brainpower. Learn the names of your participants quickly, and use names frequently. Some instructors make it a policy to give at least one correction or comment per class to each participant by name. Names have a great deal of power. Ask any salesman! Once he gets your name, he knows he has your attention. Make comments such as, "Bend your knees on this one, Sarah," or "Michael, you can do five more." Let your participants know that you are looking out for them. When you learn names, you show your clients that you think they are important.

It is best to use names during routine movement sequences or exercises so that your comments are helpful and do not interrupt concentration. Physical educators know that hearing your name called during an activity can be very distracting, especially if the activity involves coordination. Hearing your name takes your attention away from the movement part of your brain and interrupts the flow.

Tricks to Help You Remember Names

You know learning names is important, but with so many participants how do you remember them all? Practice, practice, practice! Here are suggestions from instructors:

- Review the names on your list before the first session. Of course, this only works if you have a list! If people register for your class in advance, review the list before you arrive to teach your first session. This primes those memory cells to pick up people's names a little more quickly once you meet them face-to-face.

- Give people stick-on name tags. You can do this at the beginning of a new session. Or, if your classes are ongoing, just give name tags to new people taking your class for the first few times. Make sure the names are written in big letters so you can see them from across the room.

- Take attendance. You won't learn names as easily if people sign themselves in. Some instructors check people off as they walk into the studio, checking in the latecomers at the end of class. One instructor said she takes attendance during class when people are walking around the room to cool down from the aerobics portion of class before getting weights for the strength training section. As they walk around, she checks off each person. If she doesn't know someone's name, she asks. Because it gets embarrassing to ask people their names for the fourth or fifth time, she is motivated to learn everyone's name within a few weeks.

- Give simple prizes for attending a certain number of classes. This motivates people to be sure you have checked them off on the attendance list. (This also reinforces class attendance.) Prizes can be soap, small bottles of shampoo or lotion, food, pens, shoelaces, or any little item you can afford.

- Associate an object, event, or other person with a name. It's easier to remember names if they are linked to more than one part of your brain. This means that each name is not only a word, but also has a visual image, a sound, or some other type of memory cue. Make these

(continued)

(continued)

associations as crazy as possible. Let's say you have a student named Michelle who has very curly hair. You think to yourself, "Michelle, sea shell. Michelle has curly hair like the ocean waves." Maybe you create a mental picture of Michelle as a cartoon character with her wavy hair three feet long, sticking out in every direction, picking up seashells. Write these associations on a class list (that you probably do not show your participants!).

- Use names frequently. The more you use them, the more they'll stick in your head. Greet people by name as they come into the room before class. Say good-bye as they leave. Put names on handouts, and call out each name as you hand out papers at the end of class.

- Use icebreaker activities if people need to learn each other's names. This only applies if you lead a group that incorporates time for discussion. A simple activity is to place people into pairs, and ask each person to interview his or her partner, finding out certain facts in order to introduce the partner to the group.

- If your group is very large and its members ever changing, at least try to learn the names of your regulars. Greet them as they come in to class. Ask them their names, and find out a little bit about them.

Use Positive Feedback and Comments

Give praise when people do things correctly, especially if you notice improvement or that they have corrected something. Make your comments as specific as possible. Instead of saying, "That looks good," a phrase like "Good alignment on that pose, Kevin; you've got your shoulders right over your hips," has a stronger impact. Even corrections can be phrased positively (keep your chest lifted) rather than negatively (don't slouch).

Make Comments As Specific As Possible

Many instructors limit their feedback to general phrases addressed to the whole group such as, "Good job everyone!" These are fine, but add comments that contain more specific information to make a greater impact. For example, point out to your group that six weeks ago they were only doing 8 curls and now they are doing 16. Comment on individual progress and improvement as well.

Reward Effort and Ability

People who do well or try hard appreciate being noticed. It's easiest to notice the excellent performers. But sometimes we assume they don't need encouragement. Because they look so great we assume their lives must be great. But they are really just people, and most people like to be acknowledged for their efforts. Also notice improvement and say a few words of praise to those who try hard, even if signs of progress are few.

Talk to Participants Before and After Class

Come to class 5 or 10 minutes early. As you set up, talk to the people coming in. As you check them off on your attendance list, find out about something that is important in their lives. Ask about their pets, their children, their hobbies, or their work. If your group is large or your memory unreliable, you can even jot down notes to help you remember these little details. Follow up at the next class. Ask, "How did your daughter's dance recital go? Did you get the costumes done on time?" Most people appreciate those connections that say, "Someone cares about me and my life."

Q&A

Q Don't you think that too much individual attention makes people self-conscious? I think some of my people prefer to be invisible; that's why they choose a place in the back row!

A Yes, this is a good point. Always take your cues from the people in your group. Many prefer to be anonymous in class. Instructors whose clients are well-known personalities must be especially careful to let these folks, who tend to get tired of too much attention, have privacy during class. (A well-known personality could be someone higher up in an organization who joins your class, as well as entertainment figures and so forth.) Many people want to feel that no one watches them during class. Make your connections with people who prefer privacy before or after class as much as possible, and turn off the microphone (if you use one) as you walk over to give individual corrections. How often do people want to hear their name during class? Once is probably fine for most people. So if your class is small, don't overdo the individual attention. Try to strike a healthy balance of individual attention and group flow, where people can lose themselves in the activity.

Consider E-mail Reminders

If people in your group read e-mail daily and you have a fairly stable group, ask them if they would share their e-mail addresses with you so you could notify them of changes in schedule, such as cancellations due to weather or information about registering for the next session. Use e-mail carefully and never waste your readers' time. Keep messages short and to the point.

Success Story
Keeping in Touch

The following story illustrates how a group exercise leader used e-mail to enhance the motivation of her clients. Leah started a late afternoon group exercise class in a small worksite fitness program. This program had tried for years to get a late afternoon class going at the request of several employees, but even though 20 people would sign up for the class (the required minimum), the group would quickly dwindle to about five or six participants. The class would run its course and not be offered again for several years. At this point the handful of enthusiastic employees would try again.

Leah knew the history of this class and knew that only strong motivational leadership could pull an after-work group together. An experienced instructor, Leah used a variety of activities and worked closely with the group to meet their needs. Many of her participants read daily e-mail as part of their jobs. With their permission, Leah put the group on a list and e-mailed them almost every week. Because many of her people had to reply to more than 50 e-mails a day, she kept her messages short and upbeat. She used e-mail to let people know about new things that would happen in class: "Don't forget we'll be adding weight work to the calisthenics section on Monday," or "Bring your walking shoes on Wednesday. The weather's going to be beautiful and we'll finish with a short walk on the outdoor track."

Many of Leah's participants would notify her by e-mail, at Leah's request, if they could not attend class because of illness or other reasons. She then kept in touch with them via e-mail until they returned to class. Her messages were always positive and supportive. The class has maintained its enrollment and continues to thrive five years later. All agree that Leah's motivational leadership style is the reason for the class's success.

Express Your Appreciation

People appreciate being appreciated. Never take your participants for granted. Let them know you are happy they have chosen your class. Give rewards, send cards, or have a member appreciation day. If they had not chosen to come to your class (remember, it is a choice!) then you'd be out of a job.

Your Personal Style

Personal charisma contributes greatly to a group exercise leader's popularity. Take other people's classes whenever you can and note what gives the group energy. When do the participants seem most engaged and into the class? What does the leader do to generate energy?

Personal charisma wears a million faces. Charisma can be intense and focused or playful and energetic. Develop a style that matches your personality. Without trying to be somebody else, notice what works with your groups. Express your passion for physical activity, and let your enthusiasm shine.

Nurturing Your Teaching Spirit

High-quality teaching takes a huge amount of energy. One of the most important things you can do to improve your clients' exercise adherence is to maintain balance in your own life so that you will have the energy you need to be a good instructor. Review the suggestions in chapter 1 for avoiding burnout and nurturing your creative spirit. Teach as many classes as you have the mental energy for and no more. Balance teaching with less taxing administrative or personal training work. Focus on the positive aspects of teaching and don't take dropout personally. Ignore negative attitudes; if people project negativity, it is about them and not about you. Participate in professional development activities. Make time to rest, relax, and have fun.

The "Fun Factor"

Your goal is to make exercise sessions interesting and productive, and above all a positive emotional experience. You keep your class atmosphere positive through your upbeat enthusiasm. Your corrections and comments are phrased positively. You can also help your people focus on the positive by saying, "Now for the fun part," or "Doesn't this stretch feel wonderful?" At the end of the workout you can say, "Now don't you feel great?" Send them out aware that they feel positive and energized.

Some group exercise instructors enjoy adding something different and entertaining to their classes occasionally. They might sport a costume for Halloween or use special music around the holidays. Use this technique sparingly, though. Most people don't like disruption. They want the workout they count on, so be sure that whatever you add allows the class to keep its normal pace.

Q&A

Q How do you keep your enthusiasm when you're having a bad day? Isn't it good to be honest, and if something is bothering you, let your class know you're human?

A It can be difficult to pretend everything is just fine when something in your life is really bothering you. But it is better to keep your problems to yourself as much as possible. People come to your class to feel good, and most of them have enough stress in their lives already without adding yours to the pile! Some instructors are able to admit they are under stress, let the participants know they are worried about something, and then model the stress reducing wonders of exercise by leading a great workout with cheerful enthusiasm. Other instructors say they must put their problems aside before class. One instructor remarked, "Pretend you feel great even if you don't. When you fake it, you just might start to feel better."

Welcoming New Clients to Your Group Exercise Program

Students are more open to your advice and input at some times than at others. Educators call these open times *teachable moments*. People beginning a new exercise class may present you with teachable moments. Take advantage of this openness to connect with new participants, and give them information that will help them fulfill their exercise intentions.

Can you remember the first time you attended a group exercise class? Or perhaps a time when you attended a class for an activity you had never tried before? Better yet, can you remember joining a class in a subject you had little confidence in? The first day often sets the tone for your class experience. You are relieved if the instructor is friendly and supportive and if you feel like your performance is going to be fine. You appreciate an instructor who makes procedures clear and answers your questions.

A new participant in a group exercise class can feel lost, and sometimes even intimidated. Participants look to you, the instructor, for guidance. Here's your chance. How can you make this first class a great experience? How can you take advantage of this teachable moment? This depends on the nature of your class.

Many New People Begin on the Same Day

If many new people begin your class on the same day, think about the best way to start them off on the right foot. If your entire class is new, dedicate your first class to helping them get started. If you have a mix of return and new participants, can the new people come early? Or stay for 10 minutes after class? Or can you end class early and spend the last few minutes with your new people?

You must accomplish four goals with new exercisers. First, you want them to leave after their first day feeling great! You want them to feel comfortable and welcome. Second, you want to be sure they have medical clearance to participate in your activity and can work safely in your group. You want them to be able to tell you about limitations that might affect their participation in your program. Third, you want to establish your expectations for class procedures. And fourth, you want to set the stage for good exercise adherence. To reach these four goals, follow these suggestions:

- Make it a great day. When your early birds start to arrive, shake hands and introduce yourself to them as they come in. Welcome them with a friendly smile. Give them name tags, and start learning their names. Give them the forms you need them to fill out, your class procedures in writing, and perhaps a handout with motivational reading. During the first session talk to the group about beginning a new class. Get their questions out in the open and praise them for taking this important step toward improving their health and fitness. For the exercise portion of your class, teach a simple routine that guarantees success, so that your participants walk out of your class feeling competent.

- Check medical clearance. Check over medical clearance forms, and give each person a chance to ask questions and talk to you about health concerns. Take notes on these concerns, and let people know you have heard and understood them. Above all, they want to feel safe in your hands.

- Establish class procedures. People appreciate clarity. Give each participant a handout outlining class procedures. Include information such as what to wear or where to change. Establish your expectations for attendance and procedures for notifying you if someone must miss a class. Suggest that new people stand in the middle where they can't hide but won't feel on display.

- Help people set realistic goals. Find out why people have joined your group. What are their goals? Your time for individual attention is probably limited, so encourage your participants to think about exercise goals as they fill out a goal-setting handout. Here's your chance to help them be realistic. Many people drop out of exercise programs when they discover they are making little progress toward their unrealistic goals. Usually this means they will not lose 20 pounds in two weeks as originally planned. If you have time for discussion, let the group know what kinds of results to expect from participation in your program. Emphasize improvements in mood, reductions in stress, and better sleep quality, along with physical changes such as improvements in strength or stamina.

Are people in your class new to group exercise? Some people new to group exercise may still be in the preparation stage of readiness. Help them anticipate the upcoming experience of getting to class regularly.

New People May Join Your Class at Any Time

If possible, encourage people new to your class to come early the first day. Make this a policy for your fitness center or program. If nothing else, this gives you an opportunity to review medical forms and to be sure your class is right for this person.

If conversation time is limited, can people be required to fill out a questionnaire in advance? After class? You might use this opportunity to administer a readiness for exercise questionnaire to get people thinking about their commitment to their exercise programs. You could ask them about their goals and things that have interfered with exercise participation in the past.

Use written materials to inform new people about class procedures and realistic goal setting. Provide motivational handouts about the psychological benefits of exercise, creative ideas for making exercise a priority, and other topics that enhance exercise motivation (Brehm 2000a).

Pay special attention to new people on their first day. Let them know they are working correctly or discretely give corrections. After class ask them how they feel. Do they have questions? Reassure them that they did a great job.

Q & A

Q I teach a vigorous group exercise class at a busy health club. People can join the group at any time, but my group consists mostly of clients who have been coming for more than a year. I am sure my group must be intimidating to new people, but I hate to slow down the class too much. My group really wants a tough, high-intensity workout.

A Fit people need exercise, too! It's great that your club has enough business to cater to this market. If your club offers classes for beginners and people at lower fitness levels, steer newcomers in that direction. You can still welcome new people who seem ready to take on the challenge of your class. Let them know what your class is like, and be supportive and welcoming. Once you see they have experience in your activity and the required level of fitness, give them the information they need to catch up to the rest of the class or to fit in. Reassure them that they are doing well. If you find your numbers starting to drop and you want to encourage more people to join your group, find a way to keep the intensity high but the instructions simple. This enables newcomers to adjust to your style while the old timers still get a great workout. Repetitive sequences can be simple to follow but still deliver a high exercise intensity.

Reinforcing Behavior Change in the Group Setting

Many of the behavior change techniques that personal trainers use with individual clients can be adapted to a group setting. Even if most of your group time is spent exercising, you can supply exercise adherence suggestions via handouts and one-minute lectures during cool-down or stretching. Here are some ideas for incorporating behavior change strategies into a group exercise setting:

- Self-monitoring: Self-monitoring is one of the simplest but most powerful behavior change strategies. Encourage your participants to track their workouts, including your class and any other exercise they perform. A simple one-page chart with a square for each day is sufficient. Will they turn these back in to you at some point? Maybe you can dream up a reward for people who accomplish a certain amount of exercise. Magnets to post the exercise log on the refrigerator?

- Problem solving: If you have a few minutes for group discussion, ask your participants to name barriers that have prevented them from exercising. Let the group generate possible solutions to the problems they name. Discuss challenges that may loom on the horizon: shorter days, holidays, summer vacations, or whatever might be relevant to your group. Talk about the importance of anticipating disruption and planning ahead. You can also talk about the importance of returning to exercise after being away for a while. Help participants visualize how this might occur.

- Managing stress and negative emotions: Encourage your participants to think about strategies for dealing with stress and negative emotions, so that these will not interfere with exercise adherence. Try the healthy pleasures worksheet from chapter 4. Introduce short breathing and relaxation exercises if you have time. Remind participants to use exercise to cope with stress. It's a shame that stress overload keeps so many people from exercising just when they need it the most!

- Social support: Social support improves exercise adherence. Schedule a day for your participants to bring a friend to try your class, or offer a discount to people who join with an exercise buddy.

Increasing Exercise Self-Efficacy in the Group Setting

Exercise self-efficacy increases exercise adherence (McAuley, Talbot, and Martinez 1999). Group exercise self-efficacy increases adherence to your group exercise program. What is group exercise self-efficacy? People feel efficacious when they believe they have the knowledge and skills to perform successfully in your class. Increasing self-efficacy in a group setting is not much different from working one-on-one with clients in a personal training setting. To increase self-efficacy use the following strategies to help clients acquire the knowledge and skills they need, and give them positive feedback to help them believe they are doing a good job.

- Help people be immediately successful. Present skills in a systematic fashion, letting people master easy moves before presenting more complicated skills. Give specific feedback so they know they are working correctly. Point out concrete signs of progress.

- Expose people to role models similar to themselves. Invite role models to your class to work out for free. They can show participants that people who are (pick one: old, overweight, male, and so forth) enjoy this type of activity.

- Help people recruit an exercise partner. I have discussed this strategy throughout the book. Exercise partners increase adherence in part through their effect on self-efficacy.

- Keep the focus on personal improvement. Try to eliminate competition among group members. While competition can be motivational for some, those who lose may grow discouraged. Remind your class that everyone comes in with different abilities, and the important thing is their own progress. Point out signs of progress.

Group Dynamics and Exercise Adherence

If you have led several different group exercise classes, you know that the nature of a group is greater than the sum of its parts: the individuals in the group. A group takes on a personality of its own that cannot be predicted from the personalities of its individual members. This personality has the power to motivate and enliven its members or to turn people off and keep them away.

How much can an instructor influence the dynamics of a group? Research suggests that classes whose instructors incorporate team-building activities experience better adherence, and members are late less often than those in classes without team-building activities (Spink and Carron 1993). Researchers believe that team-building activities that give a group a sense of distinction encourage a stronger group affiliation among members. For example, giving a group a distinctive name and T-shirt helps it feel special. High-quality instruction, as described earlier in this chapter, can also reinforce group distinction and encourage a feeling of cohesion among group members (Estabrooks 2000).

Other research suggests that offering an exercise class to a group with a strong sense of cohesion can enhance exercise adherence through these preexisting feelings of affiliation. In the AMEN study, researchers looked at adherence to an exercise program offered in an African American church through the African American Exercise and Nutrition project (Izquierdo-Porrera et al. 2002). Strong feelings of affiliation with the church predicted better attendance in this group exercise program than would be expected by a group without an established identity. The same kind of affiliation can strengthen adherence to activity programs in schools (for example, youth sport programs), communities, and even worksites.

Groups often take on a life of their own, sometimes without much intervention on the part of the instructor. One study by psychologist Jim Annesi (1999) found that even minimal group interaction can support adherence. Participants in his study were given standard workout programs to do on their own. About half of the participants met in small groups with an instructor for warm-up and cool-down (five to seven minutes each) at the beginning and end of the one-hour session. The participants in the control condition worked out on their own with no group warm-up or cool-down. The participants who worked in a group showed significantly better attendance and lower dropout rates than the control subjects. Annesi observed that considerable spontaneous socializing occurred among group members, and he speculated that this socializing may have enhanced exercise adherence, despite minimal group contact.

Another thing to keep in mind as you think about the groups you teach is that even though cohesive exercise groups seem to exhibit better adherence, you, the instructor, cannot always create that cohesion. While you can create a comfortable atmosphere conducive to friendliness, people have their own preferences, and groups have their own social chemistry. Forced interaction and too much attention from the instructor sometimes create social anxiety for participants.

Many people enjoy group exercise programs because they like blending in with the crowd. They do not want to think that everyone is watching and evaluating them. Rather, in a group, you expect the instructor's attention to be divided among all members of the group and the people in the group to be watching the instructor not you. When the instructor gives a lot of individual feedback, and other class members say things like, "Good job! You're really trying hard today," many people feel too visible, uncomfortable, and even anxious (Carron et al. 1999; Martin and Fox 2001). Most people want to avoid being compared to other people or evaluated on their appearance or exercise performance. That's why new people often stand in the back.

You can see why leading a group is more an art than a science. Even though most people agree on the qualities of a good group exercise instructor, when it comes to fostering group dynamics, you must often take your cues from the group members. Do everything you can to put people at ease, whether it is engaging in conversation or simply connecting through a friendly smile. Give people opportunities to connect, but don't force social interaction on people who prefer privacy.

Managing Difficult Participants

One of your responsibilities as a group exercise instructor is to deal with participants who appear to influence your group negatively. Your group exercise class expects you to be in charge. They want you to be a strong leader in control of the class. Sometimes you can prevent problems by outlining your expectations for class behavior during the first class. Or if new people continually join, you can lay out your expectations in a handout. For example, you can let people know that talking during class should be limited. Provide specific reasons for this, such as, participants must be able to hear your instructions, or injuries are more likely to occur when people are distracted.

However, negative situations can occur despite good organization. Your goal is to confront these situations quickly and decisively before they change the positive tone of your class. You can encourage problematic people to change their behavior or you can remove them from your class. Difficult people are usually easy to spot. They are often loud and rude, and usually complain a lot. When this first occurs during class, you can try ignoring them. If they are trying to get attention, they may drop the negative behavior when they find you do not reward it. If the behavior continues, speak to them privately after class. Ask if they have a problem with the class. Discuss their concerns. If the problem is something you are unwilling to change, ask them to change their behavior or leave. The good of the class should not be compromised for a few problematic individuals. Be sure to involve your supervisor if you have one. A good supervisor will come to your aid.

Success Story

Dynamic Groups

Julian, who teaches group exercise at a YMCA in the Southwest, describes a group of exercisers he inherited last year when he took over a group exercise class: "There are 10 or 12 women who have been enrolled in this exercise class for more than five years. They told me they met in class and over the years have developed friendships. They all go out for coffee together after the Friday morning class. I asked them whether the exercise instructor had anything to do with helping to form their group. They said no, she was a great instructor, but that they had gradually formed their group on their own.

"When I first started teaching this group last year, I worried that their closeness might make other students feel like outsiders, but that doesn't seem to be the case. They are mostly focused on exercising during the class, and even though they all stand together, they don't talk a lot to each other during class. I am thankful for that! Maybe one of my predecessors got them into line. These ladies give the class a cheerful, energetic feeling, and their good example of exercise adherence provides a model for other YMCA members."

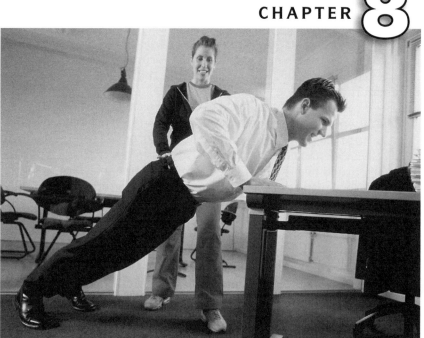

CHAPTER 8

© Sport The Library

Strategies for Fitness Centers and Health Promotion Programs

itness centers and health promotion programs come in all shapes and sizes, and can be found in an amazing variety of settings. If you are the director or are part of the management team of a fitness center or health promotion program, you are in the business of enhancing the exercise adherence of your members. (In this chapter, *members* refers to the people you serve, the people who sign up for and participate in your programs, whether or not they have joined your organization.)

As you think about exercise adherence in the context of your work, you are probably interested in exercise adherence for at least two reasons. First, you may want to help people develop and maintain a habit of regular physical activity simply because you value the benefits of regular exercise and see exercise adherence as a positive thing. Second, you may be even more interested in encouraging people to choose and use *your* center or program as a way to be physically active.

In the fitness and health promotion industries, good client adherence goes along with good business. Good business practices help to improve exercise adherence. And when you enhance the fitness success of your members, they will value your services and become more likely to renew their memberships or sign up for more of your programs. Therefore, to be successful, you must care about exercise adherence. This seems obvious, but it is surprising how little effort many fitness organizations spend on helping members develop the skills that support fitness success. You have probably visited health clubs whose primary mission seems to be the acquisition and display of exercise equipment. The priority in many clubs seems to be creating a great physical workout environment with little attention spent on helping members stick to their exercise programs.

One of your most important goals as a manager is to create the intention among all of your employees to support members in their exercise efforts. A concern for exercise adherence should have a prominent place in the mission statement of your organization. Your mission statement should express the intention to help members stick to their exercise programs and reach their fitness goals. Management must foster the belief that the exercise adherence and fitness success of each client matters. Every employee must believe that exercise adherence is the goal of your organization.

To enhance the fitness success of your clients, along with the success of your organization, you must run a well-organized business with a sound long-term strategic plan. Business advice for fitness centers and health promotion programs can be found in many places (for example, see Cox 2003; Grantham et al. 1998; Plummer 1999). This chapter highlights strategies for promoting exercise adherence in your members.

The first step toward promoting exercise adherence and member retention is to maximize the quality of your staff. You increase the likelihood that members will stick to their exercise programs when you recruit and hire great employees and continue developing current employees' exercise adherence strategies. This chapter discusses the importance of training every staff member to care about customer satisfaction and exercise adherence.

Positive first impressions increase the likelihood that people will develop the habit of exercising in your programs. This chapter discusses ideas for getting new members off to a good start and helping them through the first few months of their exercise programs. It also discusses ways to incorporate adherence strategies for new and continuing members into other programming areas.

The best way to bring people into your programs and to keep members coming back for more is to create positive emotional connections.

Your programs should be welcoming and offer immediate reinforcement through positive emotional experiences. This chapter also discusses how to cultivate positive relationships with members and how to help members experience the positive emotional benefits of regular exercise.

Fitness centers usually cater to people who are already active. However, the majority of North Americans are sedentary and overweight. If you want to expand the market for your programs, you need to reach out to these people. This chapter discusses ways to adapt your programming to reach new groups of potential members.

Quality Staff: Make Enhancing Adherence Part of the Job Description

The fitness industry has come a long way in developing professional standards for group exercise instructors and personal trainers. In the past, all you needed to get a job in a fitness center was a great body and reasonable sport or dance experience. Now most fitness professionals receive certification after studying exercise science. Many have college degrees in related fields, and some have even studied the psychology of behavior change.

Recruit and Hire Quality Professionals

A committed and inspirational staff enhances the effectiveness of any organization. Fitness centers are no exception. As you recruit people to work in your organization, look for those who love physical activity, have the knowledge they need for their jobs, enjoy working with people, and are committed to enhancing exercise adherence in your members. All of your staff members must be committed to delivering exemplary customer service and creating a positive, supportive atmosphere.

As you recruit and hire your group exercise instructors, personal trainers, and administrative staff, look for people with good communication skills. As you interview them, try presenting them with hypothetical situations they are likely to run into and ask for their responses. Are their answers thoughtful? Do they show the ability to try to understand others? Do they display a positive, productive attitude?

A fitness director at a community recreation center described an interesting job interview with a woman who had applied for a position as a group exercise instructor: "Delia's resume and application letter were perfect. She had a lot of great experience, a degree in exercise science, and the right certifications. Several of our instructors knew her, and she seemed to have a good reputation. She had cut down her teaching hours over the last several years, which is totally understandable; many of our best instructors limit their teaching hours to stay healthy and avoid burnout.

"As part of the interview, Delia taught a mock exercise class for some of the staff and me. The class was well constructed and provided a thorough workout. Delia was very fit and attractive, and a great dancer. I was ready to hire her. After the class I concluded the interview with a few more questions. I told her our numbers tended to go down in the summer. I asked her how she would feel about smaller classes. Delia responded by saying, 'I don't mind small classes, unless they are low on energy. I have a hard time when a class lacks energy. I'm tired of trying to bring people up and providing all the energy for the whole class. It drives me crazy when people drag themselves to class all stressed out and tired. I want people who come in excited to be there and happy to see me.'

"When she said that, I had to pause and regroup. Our members are like every other group of people on the planet. They have good days and bad days. Some days I am sure the group feels tired. I also know that many people say they come to class to be energized and revived. If the exercise instructor is looking to the class for her energy, we could be in trouble.

"I answered Delia's questions and thanked her for her time. After careful consideration I decided that her hope for an energetic and vibrant clientele was not realistic. We decided that Delia was not the best match for our program."

As you come to understand what kinds of people are a good match for your organization, also work toward developing diversity in your staff. Remember that potential members look for someone they can relate to. Look for diversity in backgrounds, body types, ethnicity, gender, and age. What kinds of people do you hope to draw to your programs? Can your staff relate well to these groups?

Support Quality Performance

People like to work in a nurturing, supportive environment where their efforts are appreciated and rewarded. As you structure remuneration systems for your employees, think carefully about what kinds of behaviors you want to reward. An incentive system that primarily rewards membership sales can be counterproductive in the long run. If your employees are focused on convincing people to buy club memberships, they might be tempted to exaggerate exercise benefits or promise that exercise will help clients achieve unrealistic goals. What happens when the results aren't achieved? You lose the member. Worse, you perpetuate the cycle of unrealistic promises, disappointment, and exercise dropout so pervasive in our culture.

Instead, reward excellent communication skills and the implementation and support of exercise adherence strategies. Clearly spell out these strategies, and put systems in place to monitor your members' exercise adherence. Reward employees when they contribute to membership renewals and help members reach their fitness goals.

Reinforce your organizational philosophy to support and reward customer service. Your goal is to make staff–client interactions consistently positive and supportive. Build in incentives that support this. Ask clients several times a year to nominate a favorite staff member for an award. Periodically survey members for their feedback on service quality. Ask people who participate in group exercise classes or use personal trainers to evaluate their instructors.

Use staff meetings as opportunities to develop exercise adherence strategies and to create enthusiasm for work. Provide opportunities for

Q&A

Q I have a hard time getting my group exercise instructors and personal trainers to attend regular meetings. Most of these people work part time, and attendance at meetings is usually poor. How can I get these people to attend?

A Keeping in touch with all staff members can be difficult, especially with your instructors and trainers who may work only a few hours a week. Begin by asking them what meeting times would work best for them. Maybe they don't attend because the meeting times coincide with other jobs or responsibilities. Be creative with your meeting times, and consider offering food. Some organizations find that breakfast or lunch meetings provide the best turnout. Keep meetings focused and productive. Send an agenda before each meeting so your staff will know that relevant topics will be covered. Then stick to your agenda. People presenting agenda items should be well prepared and use meeting time wisely. Look at the frequency of your meetings. Maybe if you meet less frequently, you'll have better turnout. Some organizations find that meetings with smaller groups are more focused and productive, and easier to schedule than a large meeting with everyone. How important are these meetings? If they are an important part of the job, let prospective employees know that they are expected to attend. If meetings are required, pay people to attend. You may want to reduce your reliance on meetings to communicate with staff members and look for more convenient and effective channels. But be sure to communicate regularly, not just when problems crop up. Send regular notes, memos, or e-mail to keep communication channels open. Call or meet with each employee at regular intervals to see how things are going and to let people know they are appreciated.

group discussion. Let staff instructors share ideas and strategies for motivating students, enhancing self-efficacy, or helping people set realistic goals. Provide a short reading for discussion. Encourage your staff to become familiar with stage-matched adherence strategies.

Never let your good people feel that you take them for granted. Provide opportunities for public recognition. Recognize staff contributions at meetings, in memos, and in newsletters. Acknowledge and reward excellence, such as a record-breaking class attendance, new program ideas, or solving a problem. Say thank you when an employee exerts extra effort. Pass along compliments you receive from members or other staff. Give raises based on performance.

Make everyone feel like an important part of your organization. Staff members should be knowledgeable about all of the classes and programs you offer. Encourage everyone to try sample sessions of all the classes you offer so that they can provide accurate information to prospective clients.

Support the professional development of your employees. Give them passes to visit and take classes at other studios. Fund professional development workshops. Better yet, offer the workshops at your facility—you

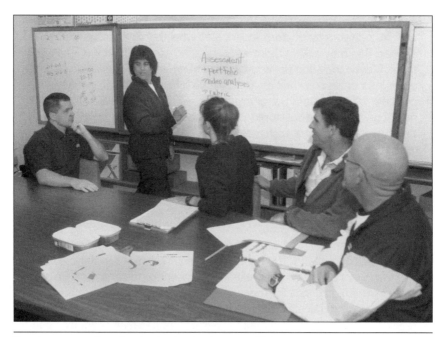

Treating your staff as the professionals they are will foster a positive work environment. It is particularly important to be organized and stay on-task during staff meetings.

usually get free passes—and encourage your people to attend. Provide financial support and time off from work if you can.

Give Members a Positive Experience

Your organization's goal is to give members a positive emotional experience each time they walk through your doors. You want them to feel welcome and at home. When a visit to your center is rewarded with positive feelings, people are more likely to come back. Their visit to your fitness center or their participation in your program should be a high point of their day. Is it?

Try to see your organization from your members' point of view, especially the way someone might see things for the first time. What are they looking for when they come to you? What do they see when they walk in the door? How are they greeted? How do they know what to do next?

The Exercise Environment

Your exercise environment is comprised of physical and social components; both are important in supporting exercise adherence. What kind of exercise environment does your facility project? What kind of clientele do you try to attract? You want to be sure that the environment feels right to your clientele. For example, if your members come to you through medical channels, such as cardiac rehabilitation, your environment should be clean and clinical. If you cater to people with families, your environment should feature family-oriented activities and perhaps child care services.

You will become better at evaluating your own fitness environment if you visit other fitness facilities. Observe your first impressions as you walk through the door and then as you tour the facility, take a class, or work out on the equipment. What does the environment say to you? Is it a "muscle-head" gym for serious body builders only? Or a rehab facility where your access to machines would be limited? Would you join this club if you were hoping to meet other young adults?

What makes a facility feel welcoming? The front desk area should be comfortable and easy to navigate, with nice lighting and decor. Consider turning off the music. The wrong music or music played too loudly can irritate some people. What works for your audience?

The most common complaints about fitness facilities are uncleanliness, broken equipment, and crowded conditions. Try to solve these problems if they occur in your facility. Find out what kinds of equipment your members and potential members are looking for and do what you can to meet their requests. What kinds of classes are most popular? What kinds of activities do people in your area enjoy?

Many clubs invest in entertainment systems that provide music and television options for clients to listen to or view while working out. Do these improve exercise participation? One study suggests that clients may exercise longer and may be less likely to drop out of an exercise program when the facility is equipped with these distractions (Annesi 2001). Consider these systems if they fit your center. Because individual preferences vary greatly, it is best to have headphones and the ability to select a channel.

What kind of emotional environment greets your members as they walk through the door? Front desk staff should be efficient, but friendly and helpful. Customer service should be their first priority. Check-in should be quick and easy.

Get New Members Off to a Great Start

One of the best ways to enhance the exercise adherence of your members is to get them off to a great start. Be sure new members receive special attention in order to help them quickly feel comfortable exercising in your facility. Even experienced exercisers can feel out of place in a new environment and appreciate guidance in navigating your facility and learning about your programs. Here are some ideas for improving the likelihood that your new members will become regular exercisers:

- The first visit should be more than a high-pressure sales pitch. Better yet, avoid the sales pitch entirely. Instead, figure out what the client is looking for, and offer advice on designing an exercise program to meet those needs. Offer a trial membership, or recommend an appropriate class or program.

- Encourage or require people new to exercise to work with a personal trainer for at least three sessions. Be sure this is convenient for the new client. The personal trainer can help clients design individualized exercise programs that address health concerns and fitness goals, and minimize risk of injury. The trainer can evaluate the client's readiness to begin an exercise program and be sure that the program matches the amount of time and energy the client is ready to spend.

- Help people experience the positive emotional benefits of physical activity. As they set goals, remind them that stress reduction is a great goal. Encourage them to look for improvements in stamina and mood, and to look for better sleep quality and less irritability.

- If you offer orientation sessions, be sure they are effective and informative, and include information on exercise adherence. People do not learn by watching; let them use the equipment with your instruction. Provide exercise logs, and handouts and advice on how to stick to an exercise program.

- Limit embarrassing and time-consuming fitness testing procedures, or make fitness testing optional. While some clients find testing motivational, people who are out of shape and new to exercise often find it discouraging. If you conduct testing, do it in private. Don't let fitness testing become a barrier to exercise participation.

- Be sure new members continue to receive helpful attention. Don't just give them an orientation session, then assume they know what they're doing. Give new members a workout card of a special color. When your monitors see those cards, they know to check in to see if the new members have questions or need help. Group exercise instructors should work closely with people new to their programs, as described in the previous chapter.

- Involve new members in the programs you offer. Give them coupons to try all of your services and classes.

- Check in with new members after three or four weeks. Ask how things are going. Answer their questions. Listen to concerns. Recommend programs to meet their needs.

Q&A

Q What do you do when you see that new members have stopped coming to your facility or no longer attend the classes or programs they signed up for? The director at the fitness center where I work doesn't contact them because she's afraid they'll ask for their money back.

A Each organization must judge the course of action that will be most productive for them. Community organizations with small budgets and a high demand for their programs usually cannot afford to spend time chasing down exercise dropouts, whose places have already been taken by other paying customers. Your director may have good reason to focus her attention on the people who attend, rather than on the dropouts. Some fitness centers find it profitable to communicate with those who look like they might be dropping out. Some organizations follow up on people who are not attending and try one more time to bring them back in. Some centers send discount coupons for their classes and for services, such as personal training sessions. Others call to say they are starting a new program that the client might be interested in. No doubt some nonattenders will mention that they are not getting their money's

(continued)

(continued)

worth from their membership. Consider waiving additional program fees or extending the initial membership period. These financial incentives will entice some people to try again. Some fitness centers send evaluation forms to people who have stopped attending to find out why. Each lapsed membership is an opportunity to learn something about your market and people's responses to your facility and programs. In an article on the importance of member retention, Darrell Cherry (2002) recommends sending a survey to people whose memberships have lapsed. He suggests using the survey to help people reconnect with their original motivations for joining your program. The survey can ask questions about their original goals and the services that attracted them to your center. Ask open-ended questions such as: "What was your reason for joining the fitness center?" and "List three fitness goals you would like to achieve this year." Promise them some sort of reward, such as free passes, for returning the survey.

Incorporate Adherence Strategies Into Your Programming

Are you doing everything you can to incorporate exercise adherence strategies into your programming? Opportunities to introduce these strategies are most likely to occur through extended staff–member interactions. For example, your personal trainers are key players in implementing adherence strategies because they work with clients individually or in small groups. Your group exercise instructors may have opportunities to reinforce exercise adherence as well. Review chapters 3 and 4 for detailed information on strategies that support exercise adherence. Some of the most successful strategies include the following:

- Match your exercise recommendations to your client's readiness for exercise. Consider the client's readiness for change. Remember that a client who has not yet made a commitment to engage in regular exercise may be overwhelmed by a complicated program. Similarly, a client without appropriate support may also be likely to falter.
- Help clients set realistic goals and look for immediate benefits.
- Set up self-monitoring procedures, such as exercise logs.
- Help clients think about ways to manage stress and negative emotions. If exercise is a positive experience, remind clients that regular exercise is one of the best ways to reduce stress and feel great.
- Build self-efficacy. Teach skills in a way that allows clients to experience immediate success.

- Make sure instructors educate clients about exercise benefits and injury prevention. Provide motivational reading on exercise adherence and successful behavior change strategies.
- Provide incentives. Reward attendance and the achievement of fitness goals.
- Encourage social support. Give discounts when members bring a family member or friend.

Keep in Touch With Your Members

Elicit feedback from your members. Listening to your members accomplishes two important objectives: You get valuable information, and they feel great. Listening does not mean you have to follow every suggestion that pops up. It simply provides useful information.

As you look at the many ways you communicate with your members and with potential members, think about the information that would be most helpful to you. Which ways of connecting with your members will offer the most representative response? How can you get the best feedback with limited resources? As you design effective communication channels, try to maximize the quality of your communication so that the process makes your members feel appreciated and heard.

Program evaluations are a good beginning. Establish procedures for reviewing your classes, instructors, trainers, and other programs. As members fill out questionnaires about the classes and programs, they are likely to answer other types of questions. For example, you could list activities you are considering adding and ask which ones they would participate in. Or ask open-ended questions: What other programs would you like us to offer? What class times are most convenient? Are you finding positive emotional health benefits from your exercise program?

Casual communication is also helpful. Hold regular member appreciation events, and serve snacks, hand out free gifts, and talk with people who stop by. Let your customers know you appreciate their business, and ask for feedback on your facility and programs.

Help People Who Are Overweight and Obese Succeed

Fitness professionals often fail in their attempts to reach people who are overweight. It is unfortunate that people who are overweight face additional barriers to exercise when they need exercise just as much as everyone else. A majority of adults in North America are now classified as overweight, and this number appears to be growing rapidly (Booth and Chakravarthy 2002). Can we afford to run programs that discourage those who are overweight?

To an overweight person, a fitness center can appear to be a temple to the sleek physique. Even the overweight clients and employees are still relatively lean compared to the general population. Fitness assessments often include measurement of body weight (sometimes in public) and body composition. Pictures of athletic models adorn the walls. The XL T-shirts are still too small.

We have studied obesity as a disease, and we are familiar with the treatment options, especially diet and exercise, but that may be as far as our understanding goes. Of course, fitness instructors and personal trainers are usually willing to help overweight clients, but may simply not know how. Many of us live in a "thin" world, often with dance or sports backgrounds and physical education environments in which few people struggle with their weight. Maybe our relationships with overweight people have been limited to advising them on weight reduction, and therefore we don't understand what it is like to struggle with excess body fat. We may have difficulty relating to them without being patronizing or inadvertently embarrassing them.

Have you ever caught yourself wondering why a fat person doesn't just lose some weight? Losing weight can be difficult for many people. Some may be genetically prone to fatness. Our culture is prone to overeating, and a history of dieting (a common experience for many overweight people) can result in additional weight gain. Weight loss programs may reinforce a negative self-image with the message, "You are too fat and you must do something about it." Dieters who fail at their attempts often lose self-esteem rather than weight. Food becomes a problem, and eating becomes an act of self-destruction or balm for an aching heart.

This is not to say that weight-loss programs always fail; some people do maintain long-term weight loss through changes in diet and exercise. But some overweight people have decided to get off the weight-loss merry-go-round, especially given the research emphasizing the health risks of repeated cycles of weight gain and loss. By focusing on fitness rather than weight loss, those who are overweight can experience the health benefits of regular physical activity, even if exercise does not lead to significant weight loss. The problem: how to get started on a safe and effective exercise program in an environment that can feel demeaning to overweight people.

Most fitness centers can increase the level of hospitality they offer to those who are overweight. Here are suggestions for improving the comfort level of your programs:

- Respect the dignity of each client. Apply the golden rule to overweight people, as you would to all of your clients. How would you like to be treated? Being overweight is not easy to hide. It's there, and it's judged. In our culture we blame people for their fatness. It is considered a sign of moral weakness and a lack of self-discipline. Respecting the dignity of overweight people means overcoming your own prejudices toward them and working with them in a respectful and professional manner.

- Don't assume an overweight person is necessarily out of shape. It is possible to be fit and fat. The overweight person you are talking to may have years of exercise experience and be quite healthy and fit.

- Don't assume every overweight person exercises to lose weight. They may exercise in order to manage stress, improve their blood sugar regulation, prevent future health problems, or just have fun.

- Don't recommend weight loss unless clients bring up this subject. People who are overweight have already been told to lose weight a million times. Like other clients, they may have special needs, such as knee problems, back problems, or high blood pressure. It may be tempting to say, "Your knees will feel better if you would lose weight," but don't. Help your client figure out an exercise program that will not stress problematic joints or exacerbate other health problems. What advice would you give a lean client with the same problem?

- Recommend appropriate classes and programs. Large people take up more space and may move more slowly than smaller people. Don't ignore their size in your recommendations. Whether an activity or class suits a particular client depends on size and fitness level. If you have enough clients at low fitness levels, consider a special class geared to this level.

What Are People Really Looking For?

People often begin exercise programs to lose weight and improve appearance. These are good reasons to exercise, but people don't need to come to your program to accomplish these objectives. What makes you special? Why should people choose your facility and programs? What is that something extra that you offer your members?

You can offer them a quality-of-life experience, a break from the routine, and a connection with others that enriches their lives. As psychologists Jackson and Csikszentmihalyi (1999, 4) point out, physical activity can offer "a state of being that is so rewarding one does it for no other reason than to be part of it." Wouldn't it be great if we could help

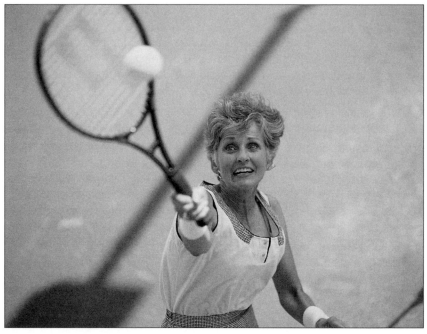

© 1998 EyeWire, Inc.

Your clients may begin a program viewing physical activity as a necessary evil for weight loss and end up viewing physical activity as something to do for its own sake—because it's fun and enjoyable!

more people experience the pleasure and recreation offered by physical activity? Inspire people to enjoy life to the fullest and to lead rich and productive lives? Part of your mission could be to provide an environment that encourages positive emotional experiences. You could offer your members a break from daily humdrum and stress, and offer them fun, connection, and even peak experiences.

Promoting Wellness in Your Community

People already committed to regular exercise make great members. They've established an exercise habit, and they generally do not require a lot of attention or support. But regular exercisers are probably a minority of your community. If you would like to expand your market, you might cultivate new programs and strategies to bring less active people into your programs.

How do you reach these folks? Some fitness professionals believe we can reach new groups of potential exercisers with a more holistic wellness approach to lifestyle change and fitness (Brown 2001). People who might not be drawn to exercise for the sake of improving their muscle tone might consider becoming more active as a vehicle to better health, stress reduction, and improved quality of life.

Thinking wellness rather than fitness can help you think outside of the box to enhance the creativity of your programming. Many people are drawn to programs that address particular health concerns. People with arthritis appreciate exercise programs designed to accommodate their movement limitations. A recent diagnosis of diabetes will prompt some to consider lifestyle change and join a program you've designed specifically for this group. More and more people are looking for weight loss success. Those with back problems need programs that incorporate safe exercise, education about ergonomics, and strategies for weight control and relaxation. When working with special groups, use a wellness approach, and combine fitness recommendations with comprehensive behavior change strategies, focusing on your clients' health and fitness concerns and goals. Include workshops on stress management, nutrition, and behavior change strategies.

Most fitness centers cater to those in the action and maintenance stages of exercise readiness. When people in the contemplation and preparation stages join a program, they often drop out because the program does not meet their needs, and they do not have the skills to maintain regular physical activity. Consider offering low-commitment workshops for people in these early stages. Discussion-based programs can help people start slowly and build skills to help them become long-term exercisers. A good source of information about discussion-based programs for people in the early stages of behavior change is the book *Motivating People to Be Physically Active* by Marcus and Forsyth (2003).

Some fitness centers increase their market share by creating lots of "entry points" into their programs. They might, for example, offer exercise programs for retirement community residents. A group of older adults might come to your facility at midday when your center is fairly empty, for a special strength training program, or perhaps the program is offered away from your facility. Either way, you start a new group of people on the road to positive lifestyle change. This program should bring in revenue and possibly create an interest in other programs you offer.

Look around your community for outreach opportunities. Consider which groups best match your interests. Schools, after-school programs, hospitals, physical therapy groups, and worksites may offer opportunities to connect with new and interesting potential clients.

Many fitness centers and health promotion organizations participate in various forms of community outreach. Some organizations participate in outreach activities because community service is part of their mission. This is particularly true of organizations that receive funding from their city or local governments. Other organizations perform community outreach as a way to create visibility for their programs and expand their markets. Participating in public service can generate free publicity and build good public relations.

We all benefit when we help raise community awareness of the dangers of inactivity. Although not everyone who decides to become more active will enroll in one of your programs, maybe some will. And then some of their friends will. By increasing people's knowledge about the benefits of regular physical activity we create a climate that is more supportive of our profession.

How do you raise awareness? What are the opportunities in your community? You might consider participating in local events throughout the year. Encourage your organization to participate in health fairs and races. Attend exercise-athon fund-raising events. Give talks at local functions and meetings. Get involved in local physical activity issues: programming at the community center or issues regarding physical education in the schools. Work with other organizations that support your mission. Create coalitions that support community-wide physical activity (Ribisl and Humphreys 1998). Lobby for the creation and maintenance of parks, hiking trails, and bike paths.

Do everything you can to build the perception in your community that physical activity must be a natural and joyful part of daily life. Help people realize that regular physical activity makes them feel great each and every day, and enhances not only their health, but also their quality of life.

Bibliography

American Cancer Society. www.cancer.org.

American College of Sports Medicine. 1997. *ACSM's exercise management for persons with chronic diseases and disabilities.* Champaign, IL: Human Kinetics.

American College of Sports Medicine. 1998. The recommended quantity and quality of exercise for developing and maintaining cardiorespiratory and muscular fitness in healthy adults. *Medicine and Science in Sports and Exercise* 30: 975-991.

American College of Sports Medicine. 2002. Code of ethics. www.acsm.org.

Annesi, J.J. 1996. *Enhancing exercise motivation.* Los Angeles: Leisure Publications.

Annesi, J.J. 1998. Effects of computer feedback on adherence to exercise. *Perceptual and Motor Skills* 87: 723-730.

Annesi, J.J. 1999. Effects of minimal group promotion on cohesion and exercise adherence. *Small Group Research* 30: 542-557.

Annesi, J.J. 2001. Effects of music, television, and a combination entertainment system on distraction, exercise adherence, and physical output in adults. *Canadian Journal of Behavioural Science* 33 (3): 193-202.

Annesi, J.J. 2002a. The exercise support process: Facilitating members' self-management skills. *Fitness Management* 18 (10, suppl.): 22, 24-25.

Annesi, J.J. 2002b. The exercise support process: The basic components. *Fitness Management* 18 (7, suppl.): 18-20.

Ardell, D.B. 1996. *The Book of Wellness: A Secular Approach to Spirit, Meaning, & Purpose.* Buffalo, N.Y.: Promethus.

Baker, R.C. and D.S. Kirschenbaum. 1998. Weight control during the holidays: Highly consistent self-monitoring as a potentially useful coping mechanism. *Health Psychology* 17 (4): 367-370.

Balady, G.J. et al. 1998. American College of Sports Medicine and American Heart Association joint position statement: Recommendations for cardiovascular screening, staffing, and emergency policies at health/fitness facilities. *Medicine and Science in Sports and Exercise* 30: 1009-1018.

Bandura, A. 1982. Self-efficacy mechanism in human agency. *American Psychologist* 37 (2): 122-147.

Bandura, A. 1997. *Self-efficacy: The exercise of control.* New York: Freeman.

Baumeister, R.F., E. Bratslavsky, M. Muraven, and D.M. Tice. 1998. Ego depletion: Is the active self a limited resource? *Journal of Personality and Social Psychology* 74 (5): 1252-1265.

Booth, F.W. and M.V. Chakravarthy. 2002. Cost and consequences of sedentary living: New battleground for an old enemy. *President's Council on Physical Fitness and Sports Research Digest* 3 (16): 1-14.

Borg, G.A. 1982. Psychological basis of physical exertion. *Medicine and Science in Sports and Exercise* 14: 377.

Brehm, B.A. 1998. *Stress management: Increasing your stress resistance.* New York: Longman.

Brehm, B.A. 2000a. *Health and fitness handouts for your clients.* Los Angeles: Leisure Publications.

Brehm, B.A. 2000b. Maximizing the psychological benefits of physical activity. *ACSM's Health & Fitness Journal* 4 (6): 7-11, 26.

Brown, P. 2001. Creating the wellness experience. *Fitness Management* 17 (12): 50-60.

Buehler, R., D. Griffin, and M. Ross. 1994. Exploring the "planning fallacy": Why people underestimate their task completion times. *Journal of Personality and Social Psychology* 67: 366-381.

Carron, A.V., P.A. Estabrooks, H. Horton, H. Prapavessis, and H.A. Hausenblas. 1999. Reductions in social anxiety associated with group membership: Distraction, anonymity, security, or diffusion of evaluation? *Group Dynamics, Theory, Research, and Practice* 3: 1-9.

Carron, A.V., H.A. Hausenblas, and D.E. Mack. 1996. Social influence and exercise: A meta-analysis. *Journal of Sport and Exercise Psychology* 18 (1): 1-16.

Castro, C.M., A.C. King, and G.S. Brassington. 2001. Telephone versus mail interventions for maintenance of physical activity in older adults. *Health Psychology* 20 (6): 438-444.

Cherry, D. 2002. Handling your atrocious attrition. *Fitness Management* 18 (1): 44-48.

Clark, N.M. and M.H. Becker. 1998. Theoretical models and strategies for improving adherence and disease management. In *The handbook of health behavior change,* edited by S.A. Shumaker, E.B. Schron, J.K. Ockene, and W.L. McBee. New York: Springer.

Courneya, K.S. and T.M. Bobick. 2000. Integrating the theory of planned behavior with the processes and stages of change in the exercise domain. *Psychology of Sport and Exercise* 1: 41-56.

Covey, S.R. 1989. *The 7 habits of highly effective people.* New York: Simon & Schuster.

Cox, C.C., ed. 2003. *ACSM's worksite health promotion manual: A guide to building and sustaining healthy worksites.* Champaign, IL: Human Kinetics.

Daly, J, A.P. Sindone, D.R. Thompson et al. 2002. Barriers to participation in and adherence to cardiac rehabilitation programs: A critical literature review. *Progress in Cardiovascular Nursing* 17 (1): 8-17.

deVries, H.A., R.A. Wiswell, R. Bulbulian, and T. Moritani. 1981. Tranquilizer effect of exercise. *American Journal of Physical Medicine* 60: 57-66.

DiBartolo, P.M. and C. Shaffer. 2002. A comparison of female college athletes and nonathletes: Eating disorder symptomatology and psychological well-being. *Journal of Sport & Exercise Psychology* 24 (1): 33-42, 2002.

Dishman, R.K., ed. 1994. *Advances in exercise adherence.* Champaign, IL: Human Kinetics.

Duncan, K.A. and B. Pozehl. 2002. Staying on course: The effects of an adherence facilitation intervention on home exercise participation. *Progress in Cardiovascular Nursing* 17 (2): 59-65.

Dunlap, J. and H.C. Barry. 1999. Overcoming exercise barriers in older adults. *Physician and Sportsmedicine* 27 (11): 69-74.

Eickhoff-Shemek, J. 2002. Scope of practice: An important legal issue for personal trainers. *ACSM's Health & Fitness Journal* 6 (5): 28-31.

Eisenberg, D. 1993. Unconventional medicine in the United States. *New England Journal of Medicine* 328 (4): 282-283.

Estabrooks, P. 2000. Sustaining exercise participation through group cohesion. *Exercise and Sport Sciences Reviews* 28 (2): 63-67.

Faden, R.R. 1998. Ethical issues in lifestyle change and adherence. In *The handbook of health behavior change*, edited by S.A. Shumaker, E.B. Schron, J.K. Ockene, and W.L. McBee. New York: Springer.

Franklin, B. 1988. Program factors that influence exercise adherence: Practical adherence skills for the clinical staff. In *Exercise adherence: Its impact on public health,* edited by R. Dishman. Champaign, IL: Human Kinetics.

Gambelunghe, C., R. Rossi, G. Mariucci, M. et al. 2001. Effects of light physical exercise on sleep regulation in rats. *Medicine and Science in Sports and Exercise* 33 (1): 57-60.

Gauvin, L. and W.J. Rejeski. 1993. The exercise-induced feeling inventory: Development and initial validation. *Journal of Sport and Exercise Psychology* 15 (4): 403-423.

Giner-Sorolla, R. 2001. Guilty pleasures and grim necessities: Affective attitudes in dilemmas of self-control. *Journal of Personality and Social Psychology* 80 (2): 206-221.

Goldstein, M.G., J. DePue, A. Kazura, and R. Niaura. 1998. Models for provider-patient interaction: Applications to health behavior change. In *The handbook of health behavior change,* edited by S.A. Shumaker, E.B. Schron, J.K. Ockene, and W.L. McBee. New York: Springer.

Grantham, W.C., R.W. Patton, T.D. York, and M.L. Winick. 1998. *Health fitness management: A comprehensive resource for managing and operating programs and facilities.* Champaign, IL: Human Kinetics.

Heatherton, R.F. and P.A. Nichols. 1994. Person accounts of successful versus failed attempts at life change. *Personality and Social Psychology Bulletin* 20 (6): 664-675.

Henderson, K.A. and B.E. Ainsworth. 2000. Enablers and constraints to walking for older African American and American Indian women: The cultural activity participation study. *Research Quarterly for Exercise and Sport* 71 (4): 313-321.

Hilgenkamp, K. 1998. Ethical behavior and professionalism in the business of health and fitness. *ACSM's Health & Fitness Journal* 2 (6):24-27, 44.

Hill, J.O. and E.L. Melanson. 1999. Overview of the determinants of overweight and obesity: Current evidence and research issues. *Medicine and Science in Sports and Exercise* 31 (11, suppl.): S515-S521.

Hospice Net: A Web site for patients and families facing life-threatening illness. www.hospicenet.org.

Hurley, M.V., H.L. Mitchell, and N. Walsh. 2003. In osteoarthritis, the psychosocial benefits are as important as physiological improvements. *Exercise and Sport Sciences Reviews* 31(3): 138-143.

Izquierdo-Porrera, A.M., C.C. Powell, J. Reiner, and K.R. Fontaine. 2002. Correlates of exercise adherence in an African American church community. *Cultural Diversity and Ethnic Minority Psychology* 8 (4): 389-394.

Jackson, S.A. and M. Csikszentmihalyi. 1999. *Flow in sports.* Champaign, IL: Human Kinetics.

Jones, F., P. Harris, and L. McGee. 1998. Adherence to prescribed exercise. In *Adherence to treatment in medical conditions,* edited by L.B. Myers and K. Midence. Amsterdam: Harwood.

Kabat-Zinn, J. 1984. *Wherever you go there you are.* New York: Hyperion.

Kabat-Zinn, J. 1990. *Full-catastrophe living.* New York: Dell.

King, A.C., C. Castro, S. Wilcox, et al. 2000. Personal and environmental factors associated with physical inactivity among different racial-ethnic groups of U.S. middle-aged and older-aged women. *Health Psychology* 19 (4): 354-364.

King, A.C., M. Kiernan, R.F. Oman et al. 1997. Can we identify who will adhere to long-term physical activity? Signal detection methodology as a potential aid to clinical decision making. *Health Psychology* 16 (4): 380-389.

King, A.C., R.F. Oman, G.S. Brassington et al. 1997. Moderate-intensity exercise and self-rated quality of sleep in older adults: A randomized controlled trial. *Journal of American Medical Association* 277 (1): 32-37.

Kreitzer, M.J. and M. Snyder. 2002. Healing the heart: Integrating complementary therapies and healing practices into the care of cardiovascular patients. *Progress in Cardiovascular Nursing* 17 (2): 73-80.

Lazarus, R.S. and S. Folkman. 1984. *Stress, appraisal, and coping.* New York: Springer.

Ley, P. 1976. Towards better doctor-patient communications. In *Communication between doctors and patients,* edited by A.E. Bennett. London: Oxford University Press.

Marcus, B.H. and L. Forsyth. 2003. *Motivating people to be physically active.* Champaign, IL: Human Kinetics.

Marcus, B.H., T.K. King, B.C. Bock, et al. 1998. Adherence to physical activity recommendations and interventions. In *The handbook of health behavior change,* edited by S.A. Shumaker, E.B. Schron, J.K. Ockene, and W.L. McBee. New York: Springer.

Marcus, B.H., T.K. King, M.M. Clark, et al. 1996. Theories and techniques for promoting physical activity behaviours. *Sports Medicine* 22: 321-331.

Marcus, B.H., V.C. Selby, R.S. Niaura, and J.S. Rossi. 1992. Self-efficacy and the stage of exercise behavior change. *Research Quarterly for Exercise and Sport* 63: 60-66.

Marcus, B.H. and L.R. Simkin. 1994. The transtheoretical model: Applications to exercise behavior. *Medicine and Science in Sports and Exercise* 26 (11): 1400-1404.

Marlatt, B.A. and W.H. George. 1998. Relapse prevention and the maintenance of optimal health. In *The handbook of health behavior change,* edited by S.A. Shumaker, E.B. Schron, J.K. Ockene, and W.L. McBee. New York: Springer.

Martin, K.A. and L.D. Fox. 2001. Group and leadership effects on social anxiety experienced during an exercise class. *Journal of Applied Social Psychology* 31: 1000-1016.

Martinsen, E.W. and W.P. Morgan. 1997. Antidepressant effects of physical activity. In *Physical activity and mental health,* edited by W.P. Morgan. Washington, DC: Taylor & Francis.

Matheny, K., D. Aycock, J. Pugh, et al. 1986. Stress coping: A qualitative and quantitative synthesis with implications for treatment. *The Counseling Psychologist* 14: 499-549.

McAuley, E. and B. Blissmer. 2000. Self-efficacy determinants and consequences of physical activity. *Exercise and Sport Sciences Reviews*: 28 (2): 85-88.

McAuley, E., K.S. Courneya, D.L. Rudolph, and C.L. Lox. 1994. Enhancing exercise adherence in middle-aged males and females. *Preventive Medicine* 23: 498-506.

McAuley, E., H.M. Talbot, and S. Martinez. 1999. Manipulating self-efficacy in the exercise environment in women: Influences on affective responses. *Health Psychology* 18 (3): 288-294.

McDonnell, A.B. 2002. Medical fitness in the U.S.: A market overview. *Fitness Management* 18 (3): 56-58.

McElroy, M. 2001. *Resistance to exercise: A social analysis of inactivity.* Champaign, IL: Human Kinetics.

McInnis, K.J. and G.J. Balady. 1999. Higher cardiovascular risk clients in health clubs. *ACSM's Health and Fitness Journal* 3 (1): 19-24.

Miller, W.R. and S. Rolnick. 1991. *Motivational interviewing: Preparing people to change addictive behavior.* New York: Guilford.

Milner, C. 2002. Why hospital fitness centers succeed. *Fitness Management* 18 (3): 60-63.

Morgan, W.P. 2000. A simple solution to the exercise adherence problem. Paper presented at the annual meeting of the American College of Sports Medicine. Indianapolis, June 2, 2000.

Muraven, M. and R.F. Baumeister. 2000. Self-regulation and depletion of limited resources: Does self-control resemble a muscle? *Psychological Bulletin* 126 (2): 247-259.

Muraven, M, D.M. Tice, and R.F. Baumeister. 1998. Self-control as limited resource: Regulatory depletion patterns. *Journal of Personality and Social Psychology* 74 (3): 774-789.

Murphy, P.J. and S.S. Campbell. 1997. Night-time drop in body temperature: A physiological trigger for sleep onset ? *Sleep* 20: 505-511.

Mutrie, N. 1999. Exercise adherence and clinical populations. In *Adherence issues in sport and exercise,* edited by S.J. Bull. Chichester, West Sussex, England: John Wiley and Sons.

Nease, D.E. and J.M. Malouin. 2003. Depression screening: A practical strategy. *The Journal of Family Practice* 52 (2): 118-124.

Nelson, M.E., K.R. Baker, R Roubenoff, with L. Lindner. 2002. *Strong women and men beat arthritis.* New York: G.P. Putnam's Sons.

O'Brien, T. 1997. *The personal trainer's handbook.* Champaign, IL: Human Kinetics.

Ornish, D. 1998. *Love and survival: 8 pathways to intimacy and health.* New York: HarperCollins.

Owen, N., E. Leslie, J. Salmon, and M.J. Fotheringham. 2000. Environmental determinants of physical activity and sedentary behavior. *Exercise and Sport Sciences Reviews* 28 (4): 153-158.

Pate, R.R., M. Pratt, S.N. Blair, et al. 1995. Physical activity and public health: A recommendation from the Centers for Disease Control and Prevention and the American College of Sports Medicine. *Journal of the American Medical Association* 273: 402-407.

Perri, M.G., A.D. Martin, E.A. Leermakers et al. 1997. Effects of group- versus home-based exercise in the treatment of obesity. *Journal of Consulting and Clinical Psychology* 65 (2): 278-285.

Petitpas, A. 1999. The client-practitioner interaction and its relationship to adherence and treatment outcomes. In *Adherence issues in sport and exercise,* edited by S.J. Bull. Chichester, West Sussex, England: John Wiley & Sons.

Plummer, T. 1999. *Making money in the fitness business.* Los Angeles: Leisure Publications.

Polivy, J. and C.P Herman. 2000. The false-hope syndrome: Unfulfilled expectations of self-change. *Current Directions in Psychological Science* 9 (4): 128-131.

Prochaska, J.O., S. Johnson, and P. Lee. 1998. The transtheoretical model of behavior change. In *The handbook of health behavior change,* edited by S.A. Shumaker, E.B. Schron, J.K. Ockene, and W.L. McBee. New York: Springer.

Prochaska, J.O. and B.H. Marcus. 1994. The transtheoretical model: Applications to exercise. In *Advances in exercise adherence,* edited by R.K. Dishman. Champaign, IL: Human Kinetics.

Prochaska, J.O. and W.F. Velicer. 1997. The transtheoretical model of health behavior change. *American Journal of Health Promotion* 12 (1): 38-48.

Raglin, J.S. 1997. Anxiolytic effects of physical activity. In *Physical activity and mental health,* edited by W.P. Morgan. Washington, D.C.: Taylor & Francis.

Ransdell, L.B., A. Taylor, D. Oakland, et al. 2003. Daughters and mothers exercising together: Effects of home- and community-based programs. *Medicine and Science in Sports and Exercise* 35 (2): 286-296.

Reed, G.R. 1999. Adherence to exercise and the transtheoretical model of behavior change. In *Adherence issues in sport and exercise,* edited by S.J. Bull. Chichester, West Sussex, England: John Wiley & Sons.

Rejeski. W.J., L.R. Brawley, E. McAuley, and S. Rapp. 2000. An examination of theory and behavior change in randomized clinical trials. *Controlled Clinical Trials* 21: 164S-170S.

Ribisl, K.M. and K. Humphreys. 1998. Collaboration between professionals and mediating structures in the community: Toward a "Third Way" in health promotion. In *The handbook of health behavior change,* edited by S.A. Shumaker, E.B. Schron, J.K. Ockene, and W.L. McBee. New York: Springer.

Riebe, D. and C. Nigg. 1998. Setting the stage for healthy living: Help clients adopt and maintain a healthy lifestyle. *ACSM's Health & Fitness Journal* 2 (3): 11-15.

Roberts, S., ed. 1996. *The business of personal training.* Champaign, IL: Human Kinetics.

Rothman, A.J. 2000. Toward a theory-based analysis of behavioral maintenance. *Health Psychology* 19 (1, suppl.): 64-69.

Salmon, P.G., S.F. Santorelli, and J. Kabat-Zinn. 1998. Intervention elements promoting adherence to Mindfulness-Based Stress Reduction programs in the clinical behavioral medicine setting. In *The handbook of health behavior change,* edited by S.A. Shumaker, E.B. Schron, J.K. Ockene, and W.L. McBee. New York: Springer.

Schlicht, J., J. Godin, and D.C. Camaione. 1999. How to help your clients stick with an exercise program: Build self-efficacy to promote exercise adherence. *ACSM's Health & Fitness Journal* 3 (6): 27-31.

Sears, S.R. and A.L. Stanton. 2001. Expectancy-value constructs and expectancy violation as predictors of exercise adherence in previously sedentary women. *Health Psychology* 20 (5): 326-333.

Smith, M.J. 2000. Clients with debilitating, progressive diseases. *ACSM's Health and Fitness Journal* 4 (2): 7-11.

Spink, K.S. and A.V. Carron. 1993. The effects of team building on the adherence patterns of female exercise participants. *Journal of Sport and Exercise Psychology* 15: 39-49.

Steptoe, A., N. Kearsley, and N. Walters. 1993. Cardiovascular activity during mental stress following vigorous exercise in sportsmen and inactive men. *Psychophysiology* 30: 245-252.

Stoll, O. and D. Alfermann. 2002. Effects of physical exercise on resources evaluation, body self-concept and well-being among older adults. *Anxiety, Stress, & Coping* 15 (3): 311-320.

Taylor, S.E., L.B. Pham, I.D. Rivkin, and D.A. Armor. 1998. Harnessing the imagination; Mental simulation, self-regulation, and coping. *American Psychologist* 53 (4): 429-439.

The National Center on Physical Activity and Disability. www.ncpad.org.

Tice, D.M., E. Bratslavsky, and R.F. Baumeister. 2001. Emotional distress regulation takes precedence over impulse control: If you feel bad, do it! *Journal of Personality and Social Psychology* 80 (1): 53-67.

Trost, S.G., N. Owen, A.E. Bauman, et al. 2002. Correlates of adults' participation in physical activity: Review and update. *Medicine and Science in Sports and Exercise* 34 (12): 1996-2001.

Turner, E.E., Rejeski, W.J., and L.R. Brawley. 1997. Psychological benefits of physical activity are influenced by the social environment. *Journal of Sport and Exercise Psychology* 19: 119-130.

U.S. Department of Health and Human Services. 1996. *Physical activity and health: A report of the Surgeon General* (S/N 017-023-00196-5).Washington, D.C: GPO.

Vasterling, J.J., M.E. Sementilli, and T.G. Burish. 1988. The role of aerobic exercise in reducing stress in diabetic patients. *Diabetic Education* 14 (3): 197-201.

Vohs, K.D. and T.F. Heatherton. 2000. Self-regulatory failure: A resource-depletion approach. *Psychological Science* 11 (3): 249-254.

Weinstein, N.D., A.J. Rothman, and S.R. Sutton. 1998. Stage theories of health behavior: Conceptual and methodological issues. *Health Psychology* 17: 290-299.

Williams, R. and V. Williams. 1998. *Anger kills: seventeen strategies for controlling the hostility that can harm your health.* N.Y. HarperTorch.

Young, D.R. and A.C. King. 1997. Adherence and motivation. In *Aerobics instructor manual: The resource for fitness professionals,* edited by R.T. Cotton and R.L. Goldstein. San Diego: American Council on Exercise.

Youngstedt, S.D. 1997. Does exercise truly enhance sleep? *Physician and Sportsmedicine* 25 (10) 72-82.

Index

Note: The italicized *f* and *t* following page numbers refer to figures and tables, respectively.

A
adherence 3-4
adherence, promoting
    exercise history, reviewing 42, 58-60
    exercise program design 60-61
    first client meeting 41-42, 43, 44*f*
    first day, anticipating 61
    fitness goals 51-57
    health concerns 50-51
    motivational approach, staging 43-50
    range of readiness 42
adherence in clinical populations
    comfort 125-126
    exercise, history of regular 120
    exercise recommendations 120
    future, planning for 124
    health problems 121-122
    logistical support 125
    pain during activity 126-127
    rehabilitation professionals 123
    scheduling convenience 126
    social support, perceived 124-125
    understanding instructions 123
American Cancer Society (www.cancer.org) 122
Annesi, Jim 157
Arthritis Today (Arthritis Foundation) 71
assessment of individuals
    action stage 35
    categorizing client 34
    contemplation stage 36
    current level of physical activity 33
    exercise questionnaire, readiness for 33
    maintenance stage 34-35
    precontemplation stage 36-37
    preparation stage 36

B
barriers to exercise, overcoming
    access to exercise 134
    depression 134
    fear of harm 135-136
    health problems and medication side effects 134-135
    low fitness levels and sedentary history 136-137
    pain 135
    self-efficacy, low exercise 136
behavior change skills
    cognitive restructuring 86-89

disorganized people 78
    exercise logs 76, 77, 78
    processes of change 80, 80*t*-81*t*
    reinforcement management and counter-conditioning 78-79
    self-management skills 75
    self-monitoring 75-77
    stimulus control 77-78
    stress and negative emotions, managing 81-86
    transtheoretical model (TTM) and processes of change 79-80
burnout, avoiding 18-20

C
career development and exercise adherence 5-7
change and people
    behavior change process 22-23
    change and adherence, stages of 40
    description of 21-22
    stage of change, assessing 32-39
    stages of change model 23-32
Cherry, Darrell 170
clients (new), welcoming
    joining at any time 154-155
    many new clients on same day 153-154
    teachable moments 152-153
clinical population, working with
    accessible exercise and special needs 114-115
    adherence 115-116
    barriers to exercise 134-137
    clinical setting 116-117
    current health trends 113-114
    exercise self-efficacy 131-133
    factors affecting adherence in 120-127
    motivational goals and behavior change skills 128-131
    settings for exercise 115
    stage theory in 127-128
    teamwork 118-119
cognitive restructuring
    description of 86
    excuses for not exercising 87, 88-89
    negative self-talk 87
    self-talk 87
communication skills
    advice, limiting 18
    connecting with client 15
    difficulties 15

About the Author

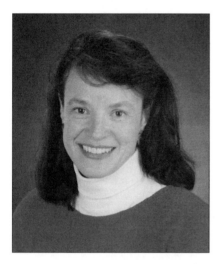

Barbara A. Brehm, EdD, is a professor of exercise and sport studies at Smith College in Northampton, Massachusetts, and has worked as a fitness instructor, personal trainer, lifestyle coach, and fitness program director. She has studied exercise motivation and adherence for 25 years and helped hundreds of people in classes and other programs become more active.

A contributing editor to *Fitness Management* since 1985, she writes a monthly column discussing recent research in exercise and health science with an emphasis on application. She has served as director of the Smith Fitness Program for Faculty and Staff since 1984. Dr. Brehm is a member of the American College of Sports Medicine (ACSM). She earned her EdD in applied physiology in 1983 from Teachers College, Columbia University.